FIT TO FIGHT

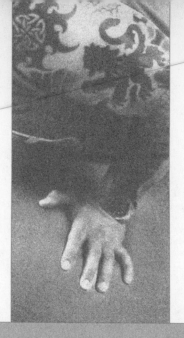

FIT TO FIGHT

An
INSANELY
EFFECTIVE STRENGTH and CONDITIONING PROGRAM
for the ULTIMATE MMA WARRIOR

■

JASON FERRUGGIA

AVERY
A MEMBER OF PENGUIN GROUP (USA) INC.
NEW YORK

Published by the Penguin Group
Penguin Group (USA) Inc., 375 Hudson Street, New York, New York 10014, USA ·
Penguin Group (Canada), 90 Eglinton Avenue East, Suite 700, Toronto, Ontario
M4P 2Y3, Canada (a division of Pearson Canada Inc.) · Penguin Books Ltd,
80 Strand, London WC2R 0RL, England · Penguin Ireland, 25 St Stephen's Green,
Dublin 2, Ireland (a division of Penguin Books Ltd) · Penguin Group (Australia),
250 Camberwell Road, Camberwell, Victoria 3124, Australia (a division of Pearson
Australia Group Pty Ltd) · Penguin Books India Pvt Ltd, 11 Community Centre,
Panchsheel Park, New Delhi–110 017, India · Penguin Group (NZ), 67 Apollo Drive,
Rosedale, North Shore 0632, New Zealand (a division of Pearson
New Zealand Ltd) · Penguin Books (South Africa) (Pty) Ltd, 24 Sturdee Avenue,
Rosebank, Johannesburg 2196, South Africa

Penguin Books Ltd, Registered Offices: 80 Strand, London WC2R 0RL, England

Most Avery books are available at special quantity discounts for bulk purchase for sales
promotions, premiums, fund-raising, and educational needs. Special books or book excerpts
also can be created to fit specific needs. For details, write Penguin Group (USA) Inc.
Special Markets, 375 Hudson Street,
New York, NY 10014.

Library of Congress Cataloging-in-Publication Data

Ferruggia, Jason.
Fit to fight : an insanely effective strength and conditioning program
for the ultimate MMA warrior / Jason Ferruggia.
p.   cm.
Includes bibliographical references and index.
ISBN 978-1-58333-304-4
1. Mixed martial arts.   I. Title.
GV1101.F47   2008   2008000953
796.815—dc22

Printed in the United States of America
1 3 5 7 9 10 8 6 4 2

BOOK DESIGN BY TANYA MAIBORODA

CONTENTS

ACKNOWLEDGMENTS

BEFORE WE GET STARTED, I'D LIKE TO THANK MY MOM, FIRST AND foremost, for all she has done for me during the last thirty-three years. While writing this book I had several other irons in the fire and was trying to do way too many things at once. The only way I was able to get through and get it all done was with my mom's help and support. Whether she knows it or not, she played a big part in this book getting finished, and for that I will be forever grateful.

I also want to thank my dad for introducing me to MMA and fitness so many years ago, setting the stage for my career.

There is another person who helped tremendously in getting this book written, and he is Sean Hyson, fitness editor at *Men's Fitness*. Whenever I needed something edited at the last minute or help rewriting a section that just wasn't flowing the way I wanted it to, I called up Sean and he was there for me every time. Without Sean's ability to simply explain what I was trying to say in much more complicated terms, this book would not be what it is.

For all of his help on the "Food to Fight" section, I'd like to thank my friend and the best nutrition expert I know, John Alvino. John's friendship and support over the last ten years have helped me accomplish more than I ever could have on my own.

I'd also like to thank my good friend Keith Scott for lending a huge helping hand with the pre-hab section. Keith's willingness to drop everything for me whenever I need it is something that I appreciate more than he knows, and I will forever be indebted to him for it.

Finally I'd like to thank my editor, Megan Newman, for being so patient with me and helpful in seeing this project through to fruition. Heaven only knows I'm not the easiest person in the world to work with. But with Megan's support (and harsh words when they were needed), the book finally got done, and I thank her for all she did in getting us there.

INTRODUCTION

I'LL NEVER FORGET THE FEELING I HAD THE FIRST DAY I WALKED INTO the House of Empty Hands in Maplewood, New Jersey. It was the fall of 1982 and my dad finally had decided to bring me to his martial arts school. He co-owned the facility with his friend and (at the time) Maplewood's chief of police, Ronny Roselli. Up until that point, my dad had only taught me martial arts at home in the basement: he had never allowed me to come down to the school to learn. When I walked in for the first time, I immediately knew why. This was not like some of the martial arts schools you see today, filled with women and children, and where contact is avoided at all costs. On the contrary, most of the students were cops or those whom the cops might be chasing as soon as class ended. The atmosphere was the definition of hard-core, and it certainly was not a place for the meek or faint of heart.

I sat quietly and timidly at the side of the room and watched the hour-and-a-half practice session. It was like nothing I had ever seen before, especially when it came time for open sparring at the end of class. The intensity was incredible and immediately I was hooked for life. From that day on, combat sports have been a big part of my life.

Although martial arts were my main focus, I began wrestling four years later at the encouragement of an uncle who was a former state champ. I had never wrestled before, but my uncle made a good argument for it, so I decided to give it a shot. I made the team, but unfortunately it didn't take long for my excitement to turn to frustration, despair, and misery. When practice officially started the next week, I found out the hard way that I was not anywhere near the shape I needed to be in to dominate on the mat.

Every day I did all the same conditioning exercises as the rest of the team. I did the push-ups, the sit-ups, the squats, and the five-mile jogs, and when I screwed up in practice I did more. I got sick and threw up often, but somehow I didn't seem to be getting anywhere. After my first season—after doing all those hours of work each week—I was nearly as weak and slow as when I started, and my conditioning still sucked.

"How could that be?" I thought. "I busted my ass!"

Eventually I started lifting weights, thinking that some strength training might help. I did what everyone else did—I used a program from a big fitness magazine—but still I got nowhere.

I'm sure many of you can relate to what I am talking about. There is nothing worse than spending hours and hours trying to improve your strength and conditioning and then having nothing to show for it when you get on the mat. The problem is that most combat athletes adopt training programs that are designed for bodybuilders, powerlifters, or other athletes. What you need is a program designed specifically for you, the combat athlete. Using the same workout that the baseball team does or something you get out of the muscle mags just ain't gonna cut it. This was the mistake I made, and unfortunately I had to learn that lesson the hard way.

When I saw my uncle again that spring after wrestling season had ended, he asked how the season went.

"Terrible," I said. "I got my ass kicked."

To this day I can remember his blank stare. It seemed like minutes passed before he said anything. And then finally he replied simply, "Oh well, you gave it a shot. Maybe wrestling's not for you. At least you tried."

What?! Wrestling's not for me? That's it?! No helpful suggestions?

That was all he offered, and I was pissed. He basically just called me a complete pussy! No one was going to tell me I couldn't do something. Now I had something to prove, and I was determined to turn my wrestling career around and become a state champ the following year. As the next season approached, I started early, doing all the exact same workouts that we used in practice every day. Just like many of you, I was determined to outwork anybody who stood in my path. I was going to show everyone what I was made of. But when practice started I still was being dominated by my teammates and opponents. Unfortunately, working hard just wasn't enough because, like a lot of you, I still was doing all the wrong things! I simply didn't know any better . . . and neither did any of my coaches.

My problem wasn't that I didn't have the skills. I actually was pretty good when we did the drills and practiced takedowns and the like. By the end of my second season the coach even picked me to demonstrate new techniques. No, technique and skill were not my problems at all. My problem was that most of my opponents were faster, stronger, and in better condition than I was. I couldn't react quickly enough to defend myself optimally, and when the tables were turned my opponents handled my offense as if I were moving through quicksand. And if I did manage to get someone into a pinning predicament, it was no use anyway. I usually was too weak to hold them down.

And my endurance?

It sucked!

You see, I wasn't born with great athletic ability. Neither of my parents were athletes. They are both under five feet six and 145 pounds. There were no gold medal-winning genetics where I came from. But I have always had an undying work ethic, and I usually could get by on that alone. No one could outwork me. But here somehow it just wasn't enough. I couldn't figure it out. I did all the recommended conditioning work and I never missed a workout. How could I be so gassed every single time I got on the mat?

I struggled through the rest of my wrestling career without ever seeing the kind of dramatic improvements from my training that I expected. I never caught on to the fact that everything I had been told about improving my strength, speed, and stamina was complete BS. I was misled for all those years, and I would go so far as to say that I had my career in combat sports ruined by inferior coaching and training methods.

Fast-forward to my college years, when I began my quest to become the number-one strength and conditioning expert on the planet. I was an exercise science major, and I was studying everything I could get my hands on about the subject. Around the same time I started taking a fighting class, which was an early form of mixed martial arts—before the sport became popular. In my studies I learned about the body's different energy systems. I also learned that most combat athletes use the wrong conditioning methods and actually make themselves slower and weaker while doing nothing to improve their staying power. I discovered how to improve speed the right way. I then was able to build up incredible strength and apply it when it mattered. And, finally, I learned the real secrets of improving my conditioning and being able to outlast any of my opponents.

I was excited and I felt invincible. I wanted to share everything that I had learned, and wanted to make sure that what happened to me would never happen to any other hopeful combat athletes. Eventually I opened my own sports-performance training facility and began sharing these secrets with hundreds of combat athletes just like you. As word spread about the results I was getting with my athletes, people began to travel from far and wide to train with me and learn my secrets of combat conditioning. Soon I had to start an application process and only accepted the most dedicated no-nonsense warriors. With every combat athlete I trained, my knowledge grew, and fourteen years in the trenches have led me to where I am today.

Now, I am going to share with you the training secrets of the world's most highly successful combat athletes. These are secrets your opponents don't want you to know.

Remember this: Even if you possess all the technical skills in the world, if you don't have the strength you need to be a champion, your career in combat sports may be short-lived. Technical skills are not always enough. In fact, statistics prove that in a match-up of two equally skilled, equally conditioned combatants, the stronger always will emerge victorious.

Unless you know how to build real, functional strength that actually carries over from the weight room to the mat or the cage, you are cheating yourself and wasting your time. But strength and skills alone are not enough. After all, what good is that strength if after five minutes you are sucking wind and completely gassed as a result of your inferior, outdated conditioning methods?

I have seen it time and time again: a great combat athlete literally having his career ruined by subpar, second-rate strength and conditioning programs.

But I'm not going to let that happen to you. In *Fit to Fight* I will help you arm yourself with everything you need to know to excel in combat sports and be able to take your conditioning to the next level.

This book is based on my years of experience, schooling, and research. It is the culmination of nearly fifteen years of hard work. The methods and philosophies outlined here are those that I have used to achieve unbelievable success myself and with countless other combat athletes. They are based on my current knowledge and understanding of the needs of combat athletes. My methods are ever-evolving, but the techniques described in this book will not disappoint. By utilizing everything you learn here, you will greatly improve your performance as a combat athlete and truly will be Fit to Fight!

FIT TO FIGHT

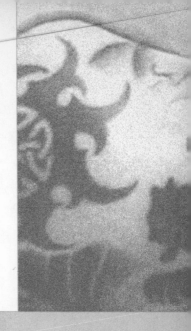

1 THE CHARACTERISTICS OF A SUCCESSFUL COMBAT ATHLETE

Mixed martial arts is the fastest-growing sport in the country, and it seems that nearly everyone you meet these days wants to get involved. I can't tell you how many times I have been at a bar or a friend's house watching a mixed martial arts pay-per-view event when someone asks me what it takes to be a successful combat athlete. Often, before I can even finish answering their question, they tell me that they have what it takes and with a little training could be the next Chuck Liddell or Randy Couture.

But do they?

Do you?

What exactly does it take to be successful in combat sports? There is a lot of confusion about this complex subject, and for good reason. A fighter needs technical skills, stamina, and strength, and most trainers can't handle the complexity of that mix. So after many years of studying and working with combat athletes, I have come up with what I believe to be the definitive training program and methods required for this demanding sport.

I'm going to outline here the characteristics *every* combat athlete must possess to achieve their fullest potential as a mixed martial artist.

Skill

The first requirement of a successful combat athlete is, of course, skill. If you are not a well-trained and highly skilled mixed martial artist, you will never be successful. In the early days of mixed martial arts most competitors came from separate disciplines with different backgrounds. You usually had a wrestler competing with a boxer or someone who studied judo fighting someone who studied Brazilian jujitsu. But as the sport evolved, the athletes realized that in order to survive and compete at the highest level, they would have to study multiple disciplines. This is why today we have mixed martial arts—where every successful competitor trains his punching, kicking, takedowns, groundwork, and submission holds on a regular basis. Basically, to be successful, you absolutely must train in some form of wrestling or grappling, striking, and submission fighting. You must maximize your training in these three areas to achieve any kind of success.

However, this book is not about teaching holds, takedown techniques, and counters. I will assume that the skill portion of your training has been taken care of and you have a qualified expert teaching you the techniques you need to improve your mixed martial arts career. If you purchased this book, you obviously have invested some time in mixed martial arts and already are training hard or are planning to get started soon. With that said, let's move into the physical attributes that make a winning combat athlete.

Anaerobic Endurance

Anyone who has ever wrestled—even if it was just fooling around in their living room with their friends—knows how draining it can be. Getting on the ground and grappling with a guy for three to five minutes is absolutely exhausting. Exchanging punches and kicks is no less demanding and also requires a great deal of endurance. This is why you need high levels of anaerobic endurance. Notice that I said anaerobic endurance and not aerobic endurance—there is a big difference, and the wrong kind of training can be very detrimental to your performance. Anaerobic means that the body is producing energy in the absence of oxygen. Most sports, with the exception of distance running and other marathon-type events, are anaerobic in nature. In fact, apart from walking, most of life in general is performed using anaerobic energy systems. To dominate your opponents and be the best mixed martial artist you can be, you have to maximize your anaerobic endurance.

To illustrate this point, picture a cheetah. The cheetah is the fastest animal on the planet. Cheetahs also are very powerful, but they have horrible endurance and get gassed in a matter of seconds. If a cheetah doesn't catch a gazelle during the first 100 yards or so, it doesn't eat, because it simply will be too gassed to keep up with the gazelle beyond that point. So the cheetah's lack of endurance actually is a threat to its survival, just like your lack of endurance will be a threat to your survival in mixed martial arts.

At UFC 22, Tito Ortiz was absolutely dominating Frank Shamrock and seemed to have the win in the bag. Then all of a sudden and seemingly out of nowhere, Tito ran out of gas and couldn't do anything but lie facedown and rest on his forearms. Unable to defend himself, he allowed Shamrock to rain down several punches on his head, at which point the ref had to stop the fight. After that, Tito swore he would never allow himself to get gassed in a fight again. So he started training at Big Bear, a high-altitude training camp, where he improved his conditioning dramatically. As a result, Tito went on a dominant winning streak and became a champion and one of the most successful and recognizable mixed martial artists in the world.

My point is that speed, power, and strength all are essentially useless without a foundation of anaerobic endurance. Looking at the animal kingdom again, think of how a good Labrador or pit bull can run around your backyard all day and then still leap into action when someone unfamiliar knocks on your front door. That's anaerobic endurance—being able to keep up a high output of power over a long period of time with little rest.

- **What are the most common weaknesses or imbalances found in mixed martial artists?**

- The most common problems most MMA athletes face are weak posterior chains, weak upper backs, and tight hamstrings. To reach the highest level, you need to address and correct these problems by strengthening the weak muscles and stretching the tight ones.

Speed

As a combat athlete, you need to be able to make quick strikes and takedowns. You also need to shoot in on your opponent quickly and make a move on him with incredible speed. You must also be able to react quickly to your opponent's actions and avoid any negative situations. So a good portion of your training should be spent on methods that improve speed and rate of force. I use short sprints, plyometrics, and medicine ball throws to help develop these skills. No matter how technically skilled you are, if you cannot demonstrate that skill with catlike speed and quickness, you are headed for trouble. For example, if you are not fast enough to sprawl when a highly skilled wrestler tries to take you down, your night could be over in a hurry. If you don't have the speed necessary to avoid a punch from a deadly striker, you could be on your back and looking at the lights before you know what hit you.

The legendary Ken Shamrock (Frank's brother) was one of the greatest fighters in the world for several years. But as he got older, he lost a step and started slowing down. The loss of speed is what ends the careers of most athletes, even more than injury. It happens in every sport. Speed is that important. Shamrock still had the knowledge and the skill (and if anything might have been even more technically sound as a result of all his added years of experience), but he no longer had the speed to compete at the highest level.

When Shamrock fought Tito Ortiz for the first time, he went in with plenty of strength, endurance, and an intense will to win, but he lacked the speed to stuff Tito's savage takedowns, or to scramble back to his feet once on the mat. Consequently, he got pummeled for three rounds, until the ref had seen enough. It was a brutal moment in the history of MMA, but the lesson was clear—you need lightning speed to defend yourself once the cage door slams shut.

Strength

Strength is only one factor when gauging success in mixed martial arts, but it is an important one. Statistics have shown that at lower levels of competition, meaning sometime before the junior year of high school, the stronger of two equally skilled athletes will have the upper hand in an amateur wrestling match and will be more likely to pin his opponent. As the level of competition increases, however, strength becomes less important and anaerobic endurance and speed take precedence. Nonetheless, it is still wise to focus on relative strength, as it can only help increase your chances of emerging victorious. At any level of competition, if all other factors are equal, the stronger athlete still will emerge victorious. Being incredibly strong can even make endurance a less-important factor—if you can manhandle your opponent early enough in the fight, you'll never really get winded. In fact, improving strength simultaneously improves endurance. As you become stronger, you will be able to do more with less effort, thus expending less energy.

The UFC's Matt Hughes has relied on his enormous relative strength throughout his career. At a fighting weight of only 170 pounds, he is known for his devastating slams and suplexes. During the bout in which he ultimately won his first welterweight title, Hughes found himself caught in opponent Carlos Newton's triangle choke. While most fighters would have tapped, Hughes mustered the strength to lift Newton off the floor and slam his head onto the mat, knocking him unconscious. The fact that many fight fans and analysts thought that Hughes had himself been choked unconscious seconds before landing the slam only serves to illustrate how strength can make the difference between a close victory and close defeat.

Flexibility and Mobility

Flexibility refers to the range of motion of muscles, and mobility refers to the range of motion of joints. Mixed martial artists need to be able to move through an extreme range of motion freely and without pain. Throwing kicks and getting out of tough situations on the ground often can test your flexibility and mobility. If you do not possess the flexibility and mobility needed to get in and out of certain positions, your chances of success are greatly diminished. One of the deadliest kicks, which ends many a fight, is the roundhouse kick to the head. You have to have great flexibility and mobility to do this. Mirko Cro Cop is a great example of an athlete who possesses outstanding flexibility and mobility, and he has knocked several opponents out cold with his roundhouse kick to the head. If you're lacking excellent flexibility and mobility, you won't be able to perform this kick, and you could tear a hamstring while trying.

Mental Toughness

This is something that you can't really teach. The psychological and emotional characteristics of a championship athlete usually are inborn or developed in the first few years of childhood. This is not to say that there is nothing you can do to enhance your potential—of course you can. If you stick a person in prison for a few years, he usually will return to society a tougher, hardened man—the environment requires it. Anyone can have his attitude changed in the right atmosphere, and anyone can develop a killer instinct if his survival depends on it. You don't need prison to develop mental and physical toughness, but you do need these attributes to succeed in combat sports. Mixed martial arts training is grueling, and the competition is even harder, especially at the higher levels. If you are not mentally tough enough to handle it, then combat sports just might not be for you. If you want to improve your chances of becoming a dominant mixed martial artist, train with the toughest group of guys around in the most hard-core atmosphere you can find. Training with guys who scare you usually is enough to change anyone's attitude.

To get the most out of your training, I recommend avoiding public gyms and either training in your garage or in some hard-core warehouse type of gym. It's important to be surrounded by a bunch of competitive guys with bad attitudes who want to train their asses off. Training among a group of guys with spiked hair and tanning cream who do nothing but curl in the squat rack is not conducive to developing the kind of attitude necessary to compete in this sport. Every workout needs to simulate fight situations in both attitude and competitive spirit.

So what exactly is mental toughness? In part it means having command over your emotions, especially fear, anger, and confusion. For the combat athlete, anger can be both your best friend and worst enemy. A certain level of anger is helpful and almost necessary—why else would you climb into the ring or the cage and try to knock out or tap out your opponent? But uncontrolled anger can result in a host of bad decisions that can lead to mistakes and your eventual defeat. This also will lead to rapid fatigue because you always will expend more energy in an angered state. You need the ability to stay calm in a fight until you see an opening, and then you must explode. Uncontrollable anger causes mistakes to be made. The best fighters are calm in any dangerous situation and are taught to always stay relaxed and loose. You simply cannot perform optimally if you are simply pissed off.

Fedor Emelianenko, the world's best heavyweight (and arguably the world's best pound-for-pound fighter overall), is known as "The Cyborg" for his incredible displays of mental toughness. Fedor has never been known to exhibit nervousness, frustration, or excitement, no matter how his fight is going—he just goes about methodically destroying his opponents. This has not only led to an awesome string of victories, but it has also added to his mystique as an unstoppable force and has made him one of the most feared fighters in the history of the sport.

That brings us to fear. Anyone who tells you he is not scared before a fight probably is lying. The prospect of having one's face kicked in will create feelings of fear and apprehension in just about anyone. But it is the ability to control these feelings that is of critical importance to the mixed martial artist. To perform at the highest level, you must be in command of these emotions and learn how to perform under extremely stressful conditions.

While some of these characteristics already may be second nature to you, you'll probably need to work on developing many of them. Remember that champions aren't born—they're forged out of years of training. Over the course of the next few chapters, you'll learn how to simultaneously develop and integrate all of these qualities to become, as they say, "a fighting machine."

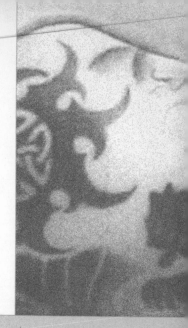

2 REDUCE YOUR RISKS: ASSESSMENTS AND INJURY PREVENTION

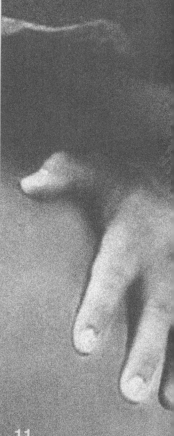

THE SECOND YOU DECIDE TO PARTICIPATE IN MIXED MARTIAL arts, you are assuming the risk of injury. It goes with the territory. Some of these injuries are freak accidents and others are the direct result of your opponents getting the best of you. In many cases, these types of injuries can't be prevented, but there are several instances in which they can be. For example, if you are strong in pressing and pushing motions but weak in pulling motions, you will be at a higher risk for injury when you throw a punch because the muscles of the upper back will not be able to decelerate properly and protect the shoulder. These types of injuries can be prevented simply by having a high level of body awareness and paying attention to the signals your body sends you.

If you have been injured in the past or are prone to injuries, the good news is that there are plenty of things you can do to improve your chances of survival in mixed martial arts if you follow a proper training program.

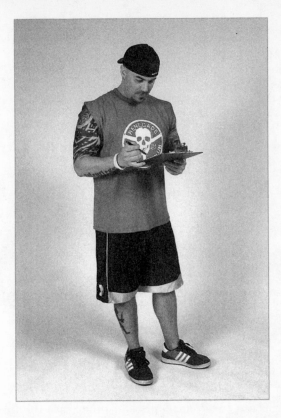

Now, in a perfect world we would all be mindful of our strengths and weaknesses and would have endless amounts of time to spend correcting our imbalances. The reality is that that's never going to happen; long assessments are impractical and often impossible in real-world situations. So I recommend a few quick, easy, and practical tests to help you get a decent idea of where you are starting and where you should end up.

The first thing we are going to address is flexibility. Contrary to what many coaches have suggested, flexibility and mobility are not separate entities. If you improve your flexibility, you automatically will improve your mobility, so in my mind the two go hand in hand. Before we go any further, I should point out again that flexibility refers to the range of motion of muscles, and mobility refers to the range of motion of joints.

TIPS FROM THE CAGE

- **What kind of warm-up should you do before MMA training?**

- I haven't included any specific warm-ups here because your coaches or instructors usually will have their own warm-ups and you will have no choice but to do them. But your warm-up should always be dynamic in nature. Avoid old-school methods such as jogging. Try a dynamic warm-up similar to the one below.

1. Jumping Jacks: 1 x 20
2. Prisoner Squats: 1 x 20
3. Mountain Climbers: 1 x 20
4. Slalom Jumps over Line: 1 x 20
5. Squat Thrusts: 1 x 10
6. Low Pogo Jumps: 1 x 30
7. High Pogo Jumps: 1 x 10
8. Leg Swings Front to Back: 1 x 12
9. Leg Swings Side to Side: 1 x 12
10. Iron Cross Lying Leg Swings: 1 x 8
11. Prone Scorpion Leg Swings: 1 x 8
12. Side Leg Raises on Hands and Knees (hip abduction): 1 x 12
13. Forward Lunge Bringing Elbow to Opposite Ankle: 1 x 6
14. Bird Dog (holding each rep for 2 seconds at the top): 1 x 6
15. Neck Flexions and Extensions: 1 x 20
16. Lateral Neck Flexions and Extensions: 1 x 20

Flexibility Tests

Testing your flexibility is a great way to determine your injury potential and find out exactly what problems are holding you back. There are dozens of flexibility tests that you could use, but I have personally found that you can gather all the information you need about the most important muscle groups and joints with just four simple tests that are described in the following section.

Overhead Squat Test

This is a great indicator of total body flexibility and, in fact, may be the only flexibility test needed, especially in limited time situations. If an athlete is inflexible in any major areas, it usually will come out in this test. Perform this test by holding a light rod or dowel directly overhead with your arms locked. From this position squat down as low to the ground as you

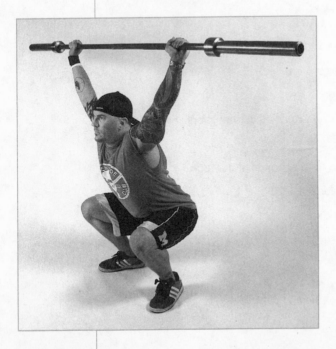

can, trying to touch your glutes to your heels. An inability to keep the bar straight overhead is a sign that the shoulders are tight and internally rotated. If this is the case, stretches for the chest and internal rotators of the shoulders must be performed regularly. You also need to do more upper back work (face pulls and rows) and less horizontal pressing (e.g., bench pressing and similar motions).

When the trunk comes forward excessively, it usually is a

sign of tight hip flexors, a weak lower back, or both. Tight hip flexors can be fixed by regularly getting into a lunge position and holding the stretched position at the bottom for 30 to 60 seconds.

If the heels come off the ground, you may have a problem with ankle stability and calf flexibility. To remedy this, stretch your calves frequently by allowing them to hang off a stair or box, while keeping your knees locked, and holding the position for 30 to 60 seconds.

Piriformis Test

The piriformis muscle is a hip rotator that can cause incredible lower back pain when tight. Having tight hip rotators will limit your mobility on the mat. Perform this test by sitting on a bench with both legs bent 90 degrees in front of you and your feet flat on the floor. Sit up perfectly straight and cross your left leg over the right. The ankle of your left leg should be just above your right kneecap. From this position, have a partner push down on the inside of your left knee. If your left leg cannot go down to a position parallel with the right, this indicates tightness in the piriformis, which can be corrected through extensive stretching. The best way to improve the flexibility of the piriformis, which will lead to increased hip mobility, is simply to perform this test on both legs as a stretch on a regular basis, holding it for 30 to 60 seconds.

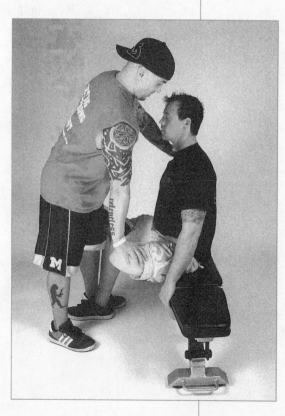

Hamstring Test

Lying flat on the ground, straighten your right leg out with the knee locked. Give your left leg to a partner, making sure to keep the right knee locked as well. The partner pushes back on the left leg while you keep the right leg flat on the floor. You should be able to get the left leg to somewhere between an 80- and 90-degree angle with the floor for optimal hamstring flexibility. If you cannot do this, you will have difficulty administering kicks above the waist and will be at risk for a hamstring pull or tear. Tight hamstrings also can cause lower back pain, which is something you don't want when you are in the cage with someone who is trying to rip your face off. To fix tight hamstrings, use this test on both legs as a stretch several times a week, holding for 30 to 60 seconds.

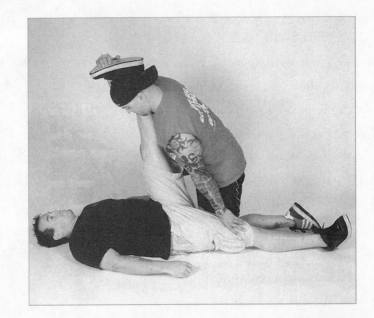

Modified Thomas Test

This is used to test the flexibility of the hip flexors. Tight hip flexors can limit hip mobility and can cause lower back pain. The largest hip flexor is called the iliopsoas. One end connects to the front of your hip and the other end attaches to five vertebrae. If the iliopsoas is tight it will pull down on those vertebrae and cause extreme discomfort. Since you cannot perform at the highest level when you are in pain or discomfort, you want to prevent this from happening.

To test your hip flexor flexibility, begin by lying faceup on a massage table, reverse hyper, or something similar. Have your glutes at the edge of the table with your right leg hanging off and your left knee pulled up to your chest with both hands. A partner pushes down on your right leg, while you keep the left knee pulled firmly against your chest. You are looking for the right leg to be able to go at least 10 degrees below the

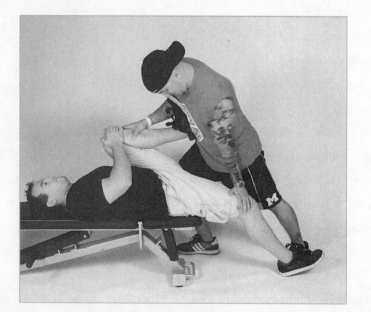

bench for optimal hip flexor flexibility. Use this test as a stretch on a regular basis, holding for 30 to 60 seconds.

Again, these tests are relatively easy to administer and can be learned quickly by anyone. Aside from these tests, I recommend that all athletes schedule a consultation with a qualified physical therapist before beginning their training.

Strength Tests

Now that we have addressed flexibility and mobility, it's time to move on to strength. With all of my combat athletes I use the following strength tests to measure progress:

1. Box Squat: 1 rep max
2. Vertical Jump
3. Chin-up: 1 rep max
4. Chin-up: rep test
5. Push-up: rep test
6. Plank: timed test

With these six simple tests I can evaluate a combat athlete's starting strength and monitor how he is progressing. I recommend that you use these tests to gauge your starting strength levels and then retest to monitor your progress every eight to ten weeks. I've chosen these particular exercises for very specific reasons, which I explain below.

Box Squat (1 Rep Max)

I use the box squat as the main lower body strength test because it is very easy to measure. There is no guessing or judgment call involved in determining whether you broke parallel or not. You simply find a box that allows you to squat to a parallel position and use that same box every time you test. Parallel means that the fold in your hips is level with your knee joints or that the tops of your quadriceps are parallel with the floor in the bottom position. While a regular squat tests leg strength, the box squat incorporates the hips to a much greater degree, which makes it a better-bang-for-your-buck test. Also, since hip strength is critically important in mixed martial arts, we want to make sure that we are improving it.

A good goal for most mixed martial artists is a double body weight box squat.

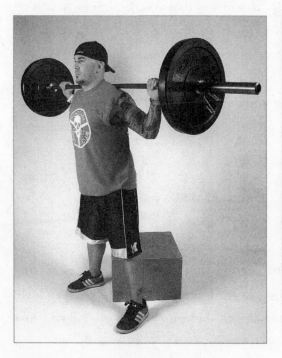 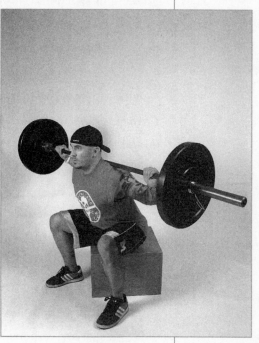

Vertical Jump

There is no greater predictor of athletic ability than the vertical jump. In MMA, a high vertical jump signifies extreme explosiveness, which translates to lighting-fast takedowns and knockouts. An explosive athlete will always have an edge over a slower competitor. The vertical jump is also a great way to measure your progress, because it tells you exactly what you are doing right and wrong with your training. If your box squat goes up but your jump doesn't, this could mean two things, neither of which is good. The first is that although you have gotten stronger, you have not learned to transfer that strength properly in an athletic way through expression of speed and power. This means that you need to focus less on strength work and more on your speed work for a while. It also may mean that you have increased your nonfunctional mass, meaning that you have gotten fatter and the noncontractile tissue is adding unnecessary weight, which is holding you down when you jump. You should test your vertical jump every four to six weeks to make sure that your training is on the right track.

A vertical jump of at least 32 inches should be your goal.

Chin-up (1 Rep Max)

Since the lats and upper back are the most important upper body muscles in MMA, I prefer to use the chin-up as the primary upper body strength test. The muscles tested with the chin-up (lats, rhomboids, rear delts, biceps) are responsible for much of what you do on the mat or in the cage. If these muscles are strong, you will be able to punch harder (with less risk of injury) and pull your opponents into certain compromising positions with relative ease. Take 1 rep max on a chin-up before you start training seriously and test again every eight to twelve weeks from here on out.

■

Look to achieve a chin-up max of body weight plus 50 percent. So if you weigh 180, you should be able to do a chin-up with 90 pounds strapped to your waist.

Chin-up (Rep Test)

While you need high levels of strength in the lats and upper back, you also need endurance. Strength without endurance is useless and will lead to defeat in a hurry. To test your endurance in these critically important muscles, I recommend that you use the chin-up rep test, which simply means that you do a set of chin-ups for as many reps as you can do until you hit failure. The total number of chin-ups you can do will not increase dramatically over the years (it's hard to do more than 20 perfect chin-ups), but it should improve somewhat. Eventually, when you can do 20 reps or so, progress will become difficult, but as long as your chin-ups are not decreasing you know you are on the right track. If everything else is increasing and your reps on the chin-up are decreasing, this could indicate that you have gained too much body fat.

■

Every mixed martial artist worth his weight in salt should be able to do at least 12 perfect chin-ups. If you cannot, you need to seriously work on improving your lat and upper back strength.

Push-up (Rep Test)

This is another great test of upper body endurance. While chin-ups cannot improve infinitely, most people can continue to increase the number of reps they can do of push-ups for quite some time. Since muscular strength endurance is actually more important than relative strength, you want to really work to increase this capacity. Testing the push-up every six to ten weeks is a good way to know whether your upper body endurance is improving.

Sixty reps should be the bare minimum number of push-ups you can do if you are serious about competing in MMA.

Plank (Timed Test)

This exercise tests the strength, endurance, and stability of the abdominal and lower back muscles. The strength, endurance, and stability of these two muscle groups are incredibly important to the mixed martial artist. If you are lacking in any of these, you will be severely limited in your ability to perform at the highest capacity and will be at serious risk for injury. You should be able to hold this position for 3 minutes for an optimal score. Once you can do that, you don't need to test this more than once every twelve weeks, just to make sure that you are maintaining your strength, endurance, and stability.

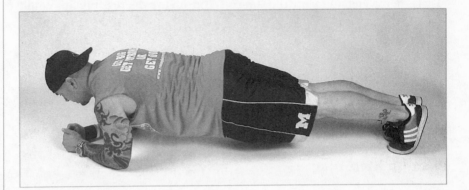

Pre-Hab

Once you have completed the flexibility and strength tests, it's time to address the common injuries in mixed martial arts. Injury prevention, or pre-hab, should be part of every serious athlete's training program. Pre-hab is an overall systematic process of preparing the body by increasing range of motion, joint stability, and so forth to help ensure that when you get caught in bad positions, you will be more able to withstand them, without injury, while stress is being placed on the joints. For example, ankle mobility will help an athlete get into better positions on the mat without injury. When you grapple or wrestle, you know you're asking your body to assume a range of motion that is way beyond normal; pre-hab will help you better deal with stress by increasing your range of motion and strength.

Before we jump into injury prevention, we need to address some potential problems. Some of the most common injuries in mixed martial arts are ankle sprains, knee sprains, hip and groin pulls, lower back pain, shoulder dislocations, shoulder sprains, neck strains, finger dislocations, and wrist sprains.

Following is a description of the most injury-prone areas and what you can do to strengthen them.

Shoulder Complex

In combat sports, and almost any sport for that matter, the shoulder area is at a tremendous risk. Think about it: You use your shoulders to grab, pull, push, and hang, all of which are possible because of the joint's tremendous mobility. But this mobility comes with a price. The shoulder is one of the most unstable joints in the body. In exchange for mobility, we give up the stability that exists naturally in many other joints of the body. Imagine moving your knee through the same range of motion as you might your shoulder on any given day. I think you see what I mean.

This lack of stability can lead to a host of problems and injuries. For simplicity's sake, I focus on two areas of the shoulder complex: the glenohumeral joint (the ball-and-socket joint in the shoulder) and the scapula, better known as the shoulder blade. These areas work together, giving the shoulder complete range of motion, strength, and stability. To protect the whole shoulder complex, it's important to supplement or add exercises into your program to strengthen weaknesses in either area, help stabilize the joints, and increase mobility and range of motion.

To keep your shoulders safe, the following exercises should be part of your training program:

Pulling Exercises. Do exercises that strengthen the back of the shoulder complex (i.e., the upper back musculature), such as face pulls, chin-ups, seated rows, and one-arm dumbbell rows.

Scapula-Stabilizing Exercises. These help stabilize the scapula and ensure normal functioning of the entire shoulder complex. An optimally functioning shoulder complex is essential for preventing injuries to that area.

Scapula push-ups are great scapula-stabilizing exercises. To perform these push-ups, get into a push-up position, with your arms straight. Now do a push-up without bending your arms. In other words, let your back sink down on the down motion, and pop up during the up motion. Remember, your elbows never bend. The motion should be slow and controlled.

Closed Chain Proprioception. Proprioception can be thought of as the language between the brain and the muscles. It's the sense of knowing where your body is in space. Imagine that you were blind and suddenly found yourself in a standing position. How would you know you were standing up? You would feel your feet compressed against the floor, as well as weight being placed on your knees, hips, and other joints. That's proprioception. Improving your proprioception will help you to have better control over all of your movements, which for the combat athlete is crucial for self-protection. When the brain and the muscles surrounding the joints work together, you'll be able to balance better, move more efficiently, and obtain stability instinctively. Improvements in proprioception make for a more efficient and better overall athlete. It also is critically important for preventing injuries. For our purposes, closed chain exercises refer to those in which at least one hand is in constant contact with the ground or is fixed while the rest of your arm is free to move. An example of a closed chain exercise is a push-up.

Alphabets are a great closed chain proprioception exercise for the shoulder. To perform alphabets, hold an end of a towel in each hand and get down on your knees. Bend over at the hips and place the towel on the floor, resting your hands on top of the towel. Keeping your elbows straight, begin tracing each letter of the alphabet with one hand and then the other. Make sure to push your hands into the floor hard so that it makes tracing the letters difficult—you should feel the muscles in your shoulders working hard. This works to fire up the rotator cuffs, the primary stabilizers in the shoulder complex that help prevent injury and increase strength. Perform 3 to 5 alphabets on each arm, pushing a little harder into the floor each time.

The next thing we need to be concerned with is dynamic stabilization training for the shoulders. The following two exercises will help improve your dynamic stabilization and keep your shoulders healthy.

Wheelbarrows. You'll need a partner for this exercise. Get down on the floor and prop yourself up onto your hands in a push-up position, with your arms straight. Your partner, who is standing, will now grab your legs. Start walking with your hands across the floor while your partner supports your legs. This exercise is a great way to dynamically strengthen the stabilizers in the shoulder complex.

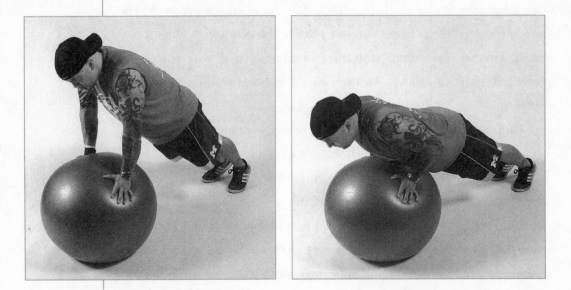

Unstable Push-ups. Perform push-ups on an unstable surface, such as a balance board or Swiss ball. Your hands are on the unstable surface and your feet are on the floor. This is harder than a normal push-up and is very good for dynamically training the stabilizers in the shoulder complex.

Hip Complex

In contrast to the shoulders, the hips generally are not so mobile. Most athletes have less-than-adequate mobility and a lot of stability—what many describe as being tight. A combat athlete must have mobility in the hips to prevent or reduce injury at and around the hip joint and lower back. At the same time, he must strengthen or activate other muscles. Some of the best exercises to strengthen the hip complex are various forms of squats (back squats, box squats, safety bar squats, and the like) and dead lifts (dead lifts from the floor, rack dead lifts, dead lifts off the mat, Romanian dead lifts, trap bar dead lifts). These will help increase strength *and* mobility at the same time when done through a full range of motion.

Feet and Ankles

The ankles are a source of a lot of misery and misconception. Most injuries to the ankles are the result of lack of mobility. The key is to increase the range of motion or mobility of the ankle joints, while also strengthening and stabilizing the inversion and eversion in the feet (turning the feet in and out). These two systems must be trained so that they learn to work together.

PROPRIOCEPTION

Ankle—Closed Chain Work.

Alphabets. You'll need a pillow, sofa cushion, or balance board of some kind for this exercise. While standing with one foot on an unstable surface and the other foot up in the air, trace the alphabet with the foot in the air, hitting all the motions along the way. Perform 4 or 5 alphabets with each foot. This exercise is guaranteed to strengthen your ankle in all directions and help you develop better balance along the way.

Eyes Closed Balance on One Leg. Closing your eyes, balance on one leg at a time, staying in the position as long as you can. By closing your eyes, your ankle and foot muscles will have to work harder to compensate for the loss of vision. Work up to about 5 minutes on each foot.

STRENGTH AND STABILITY FOR THE ANKLES

Sand Training. If you live by a beach or an area with thick sandy soil, you are in luck. Find the thickest sand possible, and with bare feet, walk very deliberately and hard through the sand, pressing down as hard as you can. Walk about 40 yards up and back. Walk forward, backward, and sideways. This training is much harder than it sounds and will help the muscles in the feet and ankles develop very quickly. Do this for 15 to 20 minutes.

Single Leg Ankle Raises. Stand on the edge of a stair and allow one heel to hang off the edge to get a good stretch in your calf. Your nonworking leg should be bent to 90 degrees. Now rise on your toes as far as you can, trying to get all the way up on your big toe. Repeat about 25 times on each leg a day.

Ankle Hops. Make a line on the floor with some tape and hop over the line, first with both feet and then with one at a time. Hop forward and backward and then side to side. Go as fast as you can while maintaining control. Do 2 sets of 20 in each direction.

Jump Rope. The jump rope may be the single best, most versatile piece of athletic equipment ever made. On top of all the other benefits (increasing foot speed, cardio endurance, anaerobic training, and coordination), jumping rope benefits the ankles as well. Jumping for just 10 minutes a day will dramatically protect and strengthen your ankles.

Wrists

Most coaches and athletes don't pay nearly enough attention to the wrist joint. The wrist is a major support for your upper extremities, and if anyone thinks that it isn't important, just try to do almost anything with an injured wrist. Taping and bracing can only get you so far. In fighting sports, you need strong, stable wrist joints to deliver effective blows. At the same time, it's extremely tough to go to the ground and wrestle when your wrists aren't working at an optimal level.

STRENGTH TRAINING FOR THE WRISTS

Sand or Rice Work. Fill a bucket with sand or rice. Plunge your hands into the bucket, then open and close your hands and fingers over and over again. This will give your wrists and forearms an incredible workout, and you will increase your wrist and forearm strength dramatically.

Rope Climbing. Rope climbing is a great exercise for any combat athlete. It helps develop wrist and forearm strength, as well as strengthen your entire upper body.

Neck

Neck injuries can be devastating for any athlete. Some are as minor as a kink or some stiffness, and others can be tragic, leading to paralysis and even death. Combat athletes need to pay particular attention to their necks. Pre-hab for this joint may be more important than for any other part of the body. Unfortunately, many coaches and athletes fail to address the neck.

As a combat athlete, you know that your neck needs a decent range of motion in all directions to best protect yourself. You must be able to move and manipulate your neck at all times in many different positions. Lack of mobility in this area inevitably will lead to some kind of trauma. Your opponent will control your neck for you if you don't. So make sure you have control. I have always told my athletes that if you can't move your neck normally, you can't protect yourself from what is coming.

STRENGTH TRAINING FOR THE NECK

Isometrics. You will need a partner for this exercise. Have him apply pressure to the top of your head by pressing down with his hands. Attempt to counter this pressure by pushing in the opposite direction. Hold each contraction for at least 10 seconds. Perform this exercise in all directions. Be especially careful training the neck—you never want to go into an extreme range of motion while your neck is under tension.

A word about loading the neck: In combat sports such as wrestling, judo, or MMA, heavy loads are placed on the spine during a competition. It is vital to have optimal strength and stability in the spine to counter the compressive forces caused by this type of loading. Some training regimens incorporate loading of the spine with techniques like neck bridging, where you balance your weight on the top of your head so your neck must work to keep you stable. This certainly will help strengthen the neck in all directions while the spine is being loaded from the weight of the body. Nevertheless, you must be aware of the potential dangers of performing this exercise and take precautions to implement it in a progressive manner. First of all, you need to have decent enough strength and range of motion all around the neck. You also must be careful not to overdo this type of training—it is my opinion that it only should be done a few times a week and for short periods of time. I have seen athletes along the way who either overdid neck bridging or were not ready for it do long-term damage to their cervical spine. Use caution with this exercise.

Knees

Knee injuries are scary and altogether too common. Ligament tears are a major concern, but stability can help prevent these tears. The best way to make sure that your knees are stable and well protected is to develop balanced strength between the quads and hamstrings. Developing your calf musculature is important as well. And good sound proprioception will help tremendously in this goal. Squats and glute ham raises are some of the best exercises to improve strength and stability around the knees.

STRENGTH AND STABILITY FOR THE KNEES:

Closed Chain Hamstring Exercises:
- Full range of motion squats
- Glute ham raises

PROPRIOCEPTION

Balance on one leg with your eyes closed. Just as with the ankle exercise, close your eyes while standing on one leg, but with your knee slightly bent. Try this on an unstable surface as well.

So there you have it—all the assessments and pre-hab exercises you need to set up an effective training program and avoid injury. With that out of the way, you're ready to start the training program.

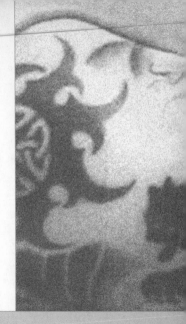

3 COMBAT CONDITIONING: BUILDING YOUR ANAEROBIC ENDURANCE

"I LOVE IT. I WANT TO SIGN UP," I TOLD OUR TEACHER, DAVID. "Okay, go down to Master Chei's studio tomorrow to pick up your gi and be here with it on for class on Wednesday."

The year was 1994 and I had just attended my first tae kwon do class in the rec center at Arizona State University. It had been a while since I had done tae kwon do, because after The House of Empty Hands closed it was very difficult to find a place with a similar atmosphere and a hard-core, no-bullshit style. I started from a very young age and became accustomed to their atmosphere and style; if I wasn't able to find it elsewhere, I would rather not participate at all.

But at last I'd found what I'd been looking for. This class was no joke, and David, the teacher, let you know up front that there were no pussies allowed and that it was going to be balls to the wall from day one. He told us that his style of teaching was to combine traditional tae kwon do with street-fighting techniques, and that we probably were going to get hurt. His words were reinforced by the bruises and welts on many of the students.

One student in particular stood out. Bart didn't look the slightest bit intimidating—he was small and kind of nerdy looking. But he limped into class the first day, taped up his injuries, and during the opening sparring proceeded to kick the shit out of everyone in his path. There were several others who seemed just as tough and well-conditioned. These were the kind of guys I wanted to train with.

I took the bus to Master Chei's the next day to get my gi. When I got there I forgot to take off my shoes, immediately pissing off the master. Then I forgot to bow, and the master was none too pleased. I told him my name and that I was there for my gi. "Dobok," he insisted.

"Great, three strikes, dummy. He's definitely gonna kick your teeth out now, you nitwit," I thought to myself.

Luckily, he let it slide and went to get my gi, er, I mean, dobok. When he opened the refrigerator, I thought he was going to offer me a beer. It was nearing happy hour, after all, and the bar on the corner had a great *Monday Night Football* party. Maybe he was getting a jump-start.

But when I looked in the fridge I found it stacked to the brim with nothing but doboks. I started to laugh like a kid in church. I knew I shouldn't have, but I couldn't help it.

"I'm really dead this time," I thought. The look on Master Chei's face told me that he didn't like me. I'm not unaccustomed to that look, but this time it was a little different. With one glance I knew that he intended to exact swift revenge on my punk ass. Luckily, he let me leave alive. Then when I walked into class on Wednesday, I again neglected to remove my sneakers. Yes, I really am as dumb as I look. "Fifty push-ups now!" David barked.

"Master Chei said you were very disrespectful."

"Way to make a first impression, douchebag. This class should be great," I thought.

For the next few weeks David punked me into the ground whenever he could and seemed to really enjoy doing so. He partnered up with me when it was time for open sparring at the end of every class. But for some reason we grew closer because of it. I think I finally earned his respect, and he definitely had all of mine.

Although I was in pretty good shape, I still was struggling to hang with the other guys in class. What I soon realized was that being in gym shape or being in aerobic shape has nothing to do with being in fighting shape. Anyone who has ever competed in wrestling martial arts or any form of MMA will tell you the same thing. All the cardio machines and bodybuilding training in the world never will properly prepare you to fight.

At the time, I didn't have a full understanding of proper conditioning methods, so I continued to struggle. Man, do I wish I knew then what I know now. I loved that class, and if I had just known how to train properly and really bring up my conditioning, I could have been so much better.

If you've ever thrown a combination of punches, kicked a bag, or taken a training partner down, you know that martial arts training tires you out fast. For that reason, combat athletes need a high level of anaerobic endurance. As discussed in Chapter 1, anaerobic literally means without oxygen, and during periods of highly intense exertion (such as throwing punches or kicks or grappling), oxygen is not the primary fuel source for your muscles. Therefore, your body, through a variety of metabolic processes, must produce energy without sufficient oxygen getting to the bloodstream. You can't train aerobically and expect to improve your anerobic conditioning—a daily ten-mile run is not the way to get yourself into condition for a match or a fight. If you improve your aerobic capacity, you do not improve your anaerobic capacity. But conversely, if you improve your anaerobic capacity, your aerobic capacity also will improve.

One of the NFL's all-time greatest running backs, the legendary Earl Campbell, used to fail his team's conditioning test every year. In fact, he couldn't even finish it, let alone pass it. Yet he was one of the greatest runners of all time. How could that be, you ask? Very simple. Football is an anaerobic sport, and most athletes run an average of four or five seconds per play, not ten to twenty minutes. The team's conditioning test had nothing to do with what Earl needed to do, namely run short distances with explosive speed. Combat sports are no different. Although most bouts have far fewer rest periods, the sport still is anaerobic by nature. And to improve your anaerobic capacity, you have to train properly. This means that the old-school, outdated approach of doing miles and miles of running each day should be thrown out the window. Not only does it train the wrong energy system, it simply doesn't work and is, in fact, counterproductive.

Take a look at the physique of a marathon runner. Now take a look at the physique of a sprinter. Which athlete looks stronger and faster? Which one looks like he would have a better chance in combat? Which one would you want to look like? Obviously, if you are going to be successful in combat sports, you would choose to look like the sprinter. The physique of the marathon runner is a product of his training. A skinny body that lacks muscle mass is the direct product of aerobic training. You do not want to step on the mat or into the cage with a marathon runner's body. And too much of this kind of training will cause you to lose muscular size and strength.

When you perform standard aerobic-type exercises, your body increases the production of the stress hormone cortisol, which is catabolic, meaning that it literally eats away muscle tissue. Excessive amounts of cortisol also make getting lean incredibly difficult. When you secrete cortisol you end up holding on to body fat instead of losing it, so you want to inhibit the production of cortisol. As a combat athlete you need to be strong, lean, and muscular. Not weak, soft, and skinny.

The Right Way

How does one go about properly training for increased anaerobic endurance? As I just told you (yet the point cannot be hammered home enough), the old-school approach of jogging mile after mile, day after day, is outdated and ineffective. Aerobic training targets the wrong energy system and does nothing to improve your performance in mixed martial arts. I'll say it again: Distance running improves aerobic endurance, not anaerobic endurance. Since all combat sports are anaerobic by nature, the inclusion of aerobic training in your workout schedule is pointless. I tried, in vain, to explain this to the father of two high school wrestlers I used to train. He was set in his old-school ways and refused to listen. When he was a young wrestler, he did distance running, so he believed that was what his kids should do. Even after I presented him with all of the facts, his mind remained unchanged. But over the summer he took his family to their beach house, and without my knowledge he had the kids run three miles every morning. When they returned home in September and started wrestling practice, he was shocked to find that the morning jogs had no positive effect on his children's performance. In fact, he told me, "They were dying on the mat today. I couldn't believe it after all the running they did all summer." "My point proven," I said.

Anaerobic training can actually improve your aerobic capacity, but as we saw in the previous example, the opposite is not true. There are few sports that require long bouts of continuous, rhythmic activity performed at nearly the same intensity. Instead, most sports require short bursts of extreme speed and power followed by a lower-intensity activity or brief rest period. Combat sports are no different, and thus the training should be no different.

Now that we know that aerobic training is useless for combat athletes, it's time to move on to what really works. Building anaerobic strength requires a multiprong approach. Since you will be participating in your sport as well as doing weight or resistance work, it's important to design a program that takes into account all aspects of your training. Plan on scheduling your anaerobic work (also called energy system work) directly after weight or resistance training, or do it on a separate day. If you are doing them on the same day, the weight training always should precede energy system training. The reason for this is that energy system work will severely deplete glycogen stores and leave you in a weakened state for your resistance workout. The goal of weight training is to increase your muscular strength, speed, and size. If you are tired and your glycogen is depleted, it will be quite difficult to get stronger, faster, or bigger, because you will not be able to give your all during the lifting sessions.

In the next section, I will outline, in no particular order, some of the training schemes that I have found to be most successful for improving anaerobic endurance in combat athletes. But before I get into these methods, I'm going to reveal a rarely used technique that I have all of my combat athletes employ. Always wear your mouthpiece when doing your conditioning drills. Breathing with your mouthpiece in is far more difficult than breathing without it. If you want your conditioning level to be at its highest when you enter competition, make sure to train with your mouthpiece in.

Finally, I must point out what may be obvious to some—that the best way to improve your endurance for combat sports is simply to fight or wrestle. It doesn't get any more "sport specific" than that. Having said that, let's get into some of the other methods of conditioning that you should be utilizing in your quest to become a dominant warrior.

Body-weight Exercises and Circuits

I routinely use body-weight exercises with all my combat athletes, usually with high reps (15 to 50) in a circuit fashion to improve their conditioning. These are some of the exercises:

Hindu Squats

Start with your hands down at your sides and your torso held erect. Descend into a full squat as low as you can go while keeping your feet flat on the ground. Make sure to maintain proper spinal curvature and keep perfect posture. When you have gone as low as you can with your heels flat, rise onto your toes and descend even farther until your butt touches your heels. At that point, lift your arms out straight in front of you. Extend your hips and knees to return to the starting position.

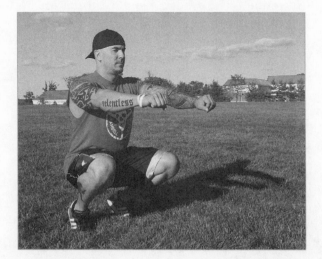

Prisoner Squats

Start with your hands clasped behind your head in a perfectly upright posture. Squat straight down as low as you can while maintaining perfect posture, keeping your heels flat on the ground. Extend your hips and knees to return to the starting position.

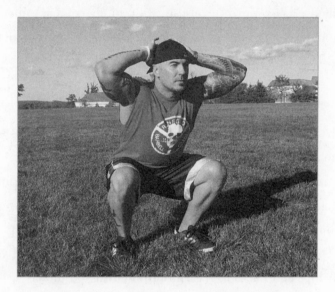

Hindu Push-ups

Start in a normal push-up position, and from there walk your feet forward until your body is in an A-frame position, with your butt held high in the air. Begin the descent by diving straight down toward the floor and skimming it with your chest. Continue in an arclike motion and keep going forward until your hips are nearly even with your hands. As you start to come up, look toward the ceiling. From this position, drop your head, raise your butt back up to the starting position, and repeat.

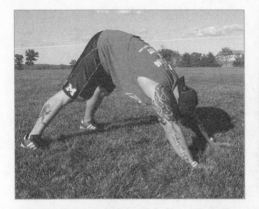
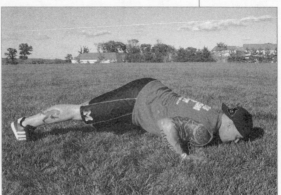

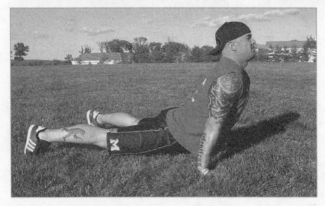

Forward Lunges

The standard lunge, performed with both hands on your hips. Step forward as far as you can while maintaining a perfectly upright posture before explosively pushing yourself back to the starting position and switching legs. Make sure to get a good stretch in the hip flexors.

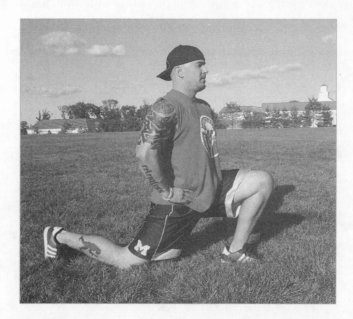

Reverse Lunges

The opposite of the forward lunge. Start by stepping backward and descending into the full lunge position. Return to the starting position and switch legs.

Jumping Lunges

Start in a forward lunge position and jump as high as you can while simultaneously switching your feet in midair.

Bootstrappers

With your feet flat on the floor, bend down and grab the front of your sneakers under your toes (if you have poor flexibility you can hold on to the tongue of your sneakers instead). From this position, descend into a full squat while keeping your hands on the floor. Remaining in this bent-over position, blast back up until your legs are a few inches shy of being locked out completely. This is an important point to remember, because this is meant to be more of a quadriceps exercise than a hamstring stretch, so you want to maintain a slight knee bend and keep constant tension on your quads.

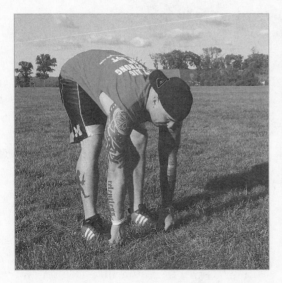 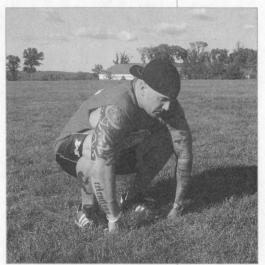

Mountain Climbers

Start in a push-up position. Begin by bringing one knee to your chest and then as you return that leg to the starting position, bring the opposite leg up. This should be performed at a quick pace—think of running in place while in a push-up position.

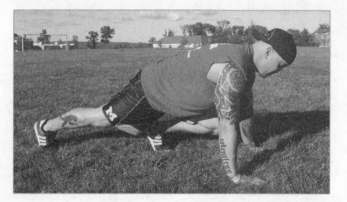

Grasshoppers

Start in a push-up position. From there, rotate your hips to the left, bringing your left leg underneath your right and kicking it straight out to your right side. Immediately switch sides and kick your right leg out to your left side.

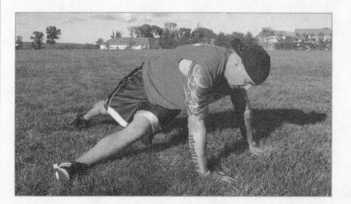

Bear Walks

Get down with your hands flat on the ground and simply walk around like a bear on your hands and feet. This should be performed for distance, such as from one side of the gym to the other, or better yet, outside on a field. Ideally, you want to have at least a 50-foot straightaway to do these. To increase the difficulty, you can attach a weighted sled to a belt tied around your waist or to each ankle.

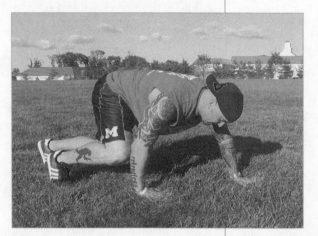

Duck Walks

Squat down as low as you can and walk forward in this position for 50 to 100 feet.

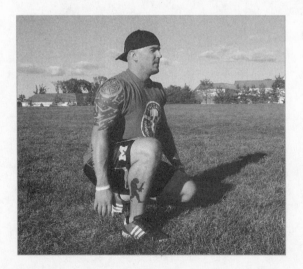

Crab Walks

Sitting on the floor, place your hands underneath yourself and raise your body to a position parallel with the ground. Think of your body as a table, with your chest and belly as the tabletop. Keep your knees bent at 90 degrees. Walk for 50 to 100 feet in this position while keeping your hips up and body straight in line.

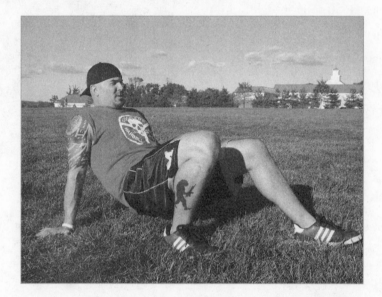

Wheelbarrow Walks

You will need a partner for this one. Begin in a push-up position and have your partner hold your legs. Using your arms, walk forward for 50 to 100 feet, making sure not to let your hips sag or rotate excessively.

Jumping Jacks

No description necessary.

Ali Shuffle

With hands on hips, shuffle your feet forward and backward rapidly, making sure to maintain perfect posture.

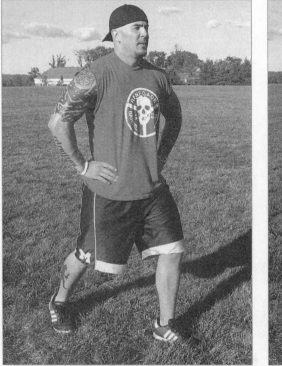 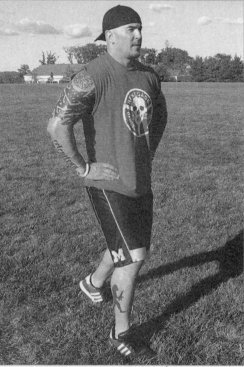

Shuffle Jacks

Performed like standard jumping jacks but with your feet moving forward and backward as in the Ali shuffle.

Seal Jumps

Similar to jumping jacks, but instead of raising your arms overhead, you reach them straight out to your sides, stretching your chest. As your legs come back together (as in the jumping jack), you clap your hands together like a seal.

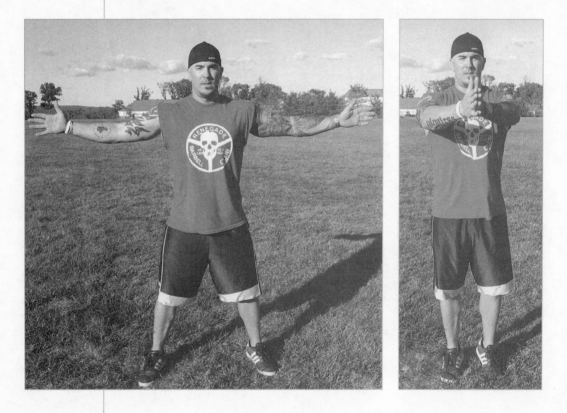

Slalom Jumps

With your hands on your hips, jump side to side over an imaginary line or small hurdle. Make sure to keep ground contact time minimal.

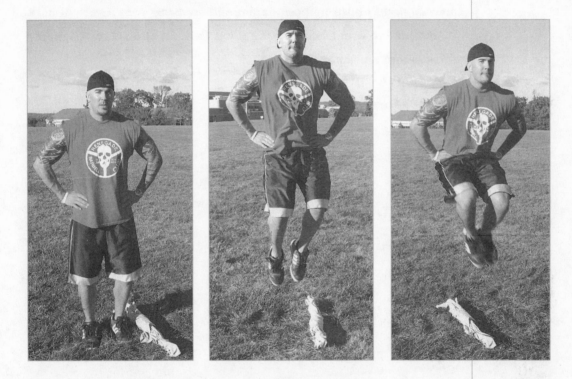

Squat Thrusts

Standing with your hands at your sides, squat down and place your hands on the floor. Immediately shoot your legs straight out so that you are in a perfect push-up position. From there bring your legs right back in and pick your hands up off the floor. Perform an explosive jumping squat before repeating.

Step-ups

You'll need a box or bleacher seat for this exercise. With both feet flat on the floor, take one leg and step up onto a box or bleacher seat. Make sure that you are only using the stepping leg to hoist yourself onto the box. Return to the starting position and repeat with the other leg.

Reverse Push-ups

Start by lying on your back with your feet flat on the floor. Place your hands beside your ears with your palms on the ground. From this position, push yourself up into a full bridge by extending your arms and legs. This

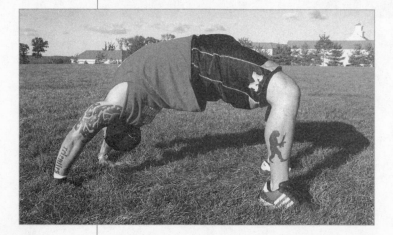

exercise can be done for time or for reps—for example, you can hold it in the top position as long as possible or bend your elbows and lower your body closer to the floor and then push back up (1 rep).

Tabletops

While sitting on the ground, place your hands and feet flat on the floor. Rise up until your legs are bent 90 degrees and your arms are straight. Completely straighten out your torso (the tabletop) and hold this position. This should be done for time and not reps—simply hold the position as long as you can.

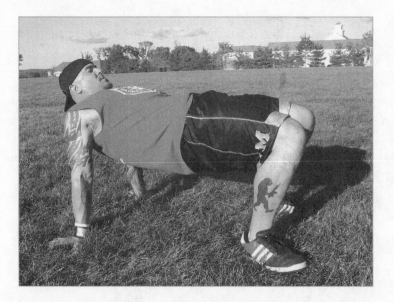

Side Outs

Begin with your hands flat on the ground and your knees bent 90 degrees. Shoot your legs out to one side while simultaneously raising the hand on the same side off the ground and supporting all your weight on the other arm. Immediately reverse directions and repeat on the other side.

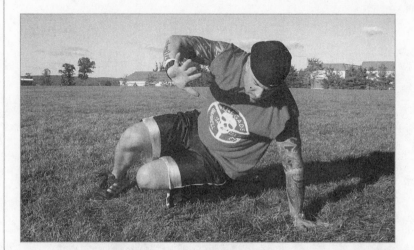

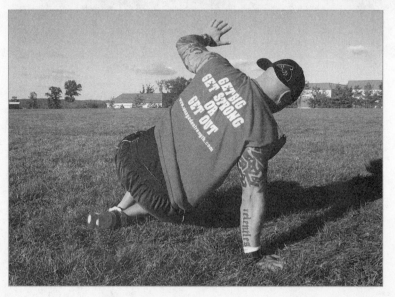

Push-ups

No description necessary.

Sit-ups

These body-weight exercises are great for all combat athletes and can be included in your training program in a variety of ways. One way, as mentioned earlier, is to use them in a moderate-rep to high-rep circuit. You can do this at the end of a regular strength-training workout or on a separate day dedicated solely to conditioning. Coaches may also incorporate these exercises into their practice sessions. They can be done as warm-ups and/or as a good finisher after practice. I normally do four to six exercises and perform them in a circuit fashion for five to seven rounds with minimal rest periods. As your conditioning improves, increase the number of reps or sets performed or try to complete the same number of sets and reps in less time than your previous workout. Below is an example of an effective body-weight circuit routine. Beware—these circuits will be much harder than they look the first few times you do them.

1. Prisoner Squats: 50 reps
2. Hindu Push-ups: 25 reps
3. Mountain Climbers: 60 seconds
4. Reverse Push-ups: 60 seconds
5. Side Outs: 60 seconds

Again, this is only one way of using these exercises. Basically, you want to pick some kind of lower body exercise, an upper body exercise, a jumping exercise, a bridging exercise, and a jumping exercise, and put them together in a circuit.

Another example:

1. Squat Thrusts: 15 reps
2. Reverse Push-ups: hold as long as possible
3. Slalom Jumps: 60 seconds
4. Bear Walks: 50 yards
5. Bootstrappers: 25 reps
6. Shuffle Jacks: 60 seconds

If you get creative, you can come up with infinite ways of incorporating these exercises into your training program.

For advanced athletes, try using a weighted vest for some of the exercises. I do this with my combat athletes, as the weight of the vest simulates competition. As you know, when you are on the mat, many of the moves you make will be done with the weight of your competitor on you in some way or another. So the weighted vest helps you get used to moving with this burden. The key is not to let your exercise form get sloppy or slow. You want to select a weight that is heavy enough to challenge you yet light enough to still allow you to do the drills in perfect form and without any loss of speed or power.

Sprints

While jogging is a complete waste of time for combat athletes, sprinting is one of the best forms of exercise you can do. Sprinting will work wonders for your anaerobic capacity and get you in tremendous shape. I have all my combat athletes on a strict sprinting regimen. The types of sprinting workouts vary greatly from one training session to the next. Here are some of my favorite sprint workouts:

Intervals

These sessions usually involve sprinting for 10 to 15 seconds, followed by a slower-paced jog or walk of 30 to 90 seconds. You could go to a track and sprint the length of the straightaway and walk the curves, then repeat for 8 to 10 sets. You don't want to run 100 percent all out during these intervals, more like 80 to 85 precent. If you've never run sprints before, this can be an incredibly grueling workout, so pace yourself. Another option is to run shorter sprints of 40 to 50 yards and simply walk back to the starting position before repeating. This is not the best way to develop maximal speed, but it is excellent for conditioning.

Hill Sprints

This is an extremely difficult yet incredibly effective exercise for combat athletes. You'll need to find a 50- to 100-yard hill. Sprint up, walk down, then repeat. Your rest between sprints should be minimal. As the sprints get easier, decrease your rest periods—this way you are performing more work in a given amount of time. Surprisingly, hill sprints are safer than flat ground sprints, especially for those not used to sprinting. Because you won't be able to run them terribly fast, you are less likely to get injured, say by pulling a hamstring or straining a hip flexor. Hill running also places less strain on all of your joints. So despite the pain, there are lots of advantages to running hills.

Sled Sprints

Sprinting with a sled is another great way of increasing your conditioning. A dragging sled is a platform with a rope or handle attachment that you can pile weights on (you can also use it as is). You can tie it around your waist or hold the handles to perform numerous exercises, including forward and backward sprints. Like sprinting on a hill, the sled will slow you down and help you avoid any possible hamstring or hip flexor injuries. Another benefit to using the sled is that you can add weight to it and build strength, speed, and endurance all with one implement. To use the sled optimally, you'll need a field with at least a 100-foot straightaway. I prefer to do 30- to 40-yard sprints with the sled, alternating between backward and forward sprints every other set. You can get a great dragging sled at EliteFTS.com.

300-Yard Shuttle Runs

Many football players get tested in the 300-yard shuttle during preseason training camp. It is also a great way for the combat athlete to bring up his conditioning. There are two ways to do the 300-yard shuttle. One is to set cones 25 yards apart and sprint back and forth 12 times. Another is to set the cones 50 yards apart and sprint back and forth 6 times. After each shuttle, rest a minute or so and repeat for 3 to 4 sets.

Stadium Stair Sprints

This one is pretty self-explanatory. You go down to the local high school or college field and sprint up the stadium stairs. This is one of the oldest methods in the book when it comes to conditioning but also one of the most effective. The interval pattern you use will depend on the length of the stairs. If the stairs are longer, you may want to sprint straight up, walk back down, and repeat for 12 to 15 sets. If the stairs are a bit shorter, you could sprint up, jog down, and repeat 4 or 5 times before taking a short (60- to 90-second) rest period before returning for another 8 to 10 sets.

Agility Circuits

Although not "sport specific" for the combat athlete, running agility circuits is a great way to improve your conditioning rapidly. By agility circuits, I mean a group of exercises that improve your ability to rapidly change direction. These circuits should last between 10 and 60 seconds, depending on your level of conditioning. An example of an agility circuit is to set up 4 cones in a square about 20 to 30 feet apart. Sprint straight ahead to the first cone and touch it, side shuffle to the next cone and touch it, back-peddle to the next cone and touch it, side shuffle to the last cone and touch it, rest, and repeat. Another option is to add in some low hurdles. You could start by jumping sideways over 6 low hurdles, then sprinting straight ahead to the next set of hurdles and jumping sideways over them, followed by a backward sprint to the finish. If you use your imagination, you can come up with an infinite number of agility circuits.

Medicine Ball Throw and Retrieve

This is a great way to simultaneously train for explosive speed and anaerobic endurance. Simply scoop a medicine ball off the floor and throw it as hard as you can forward or backward over your head, and sprint to retrieve it. Use a fairly light ball that you can throw a good distance (obviously, this drill should be done outside in a wide-open area). Do 6 throws and then rest for a minute before repeating. Do 8 to 10 rounds.

Barbell Complexes

Barbell complexes are a great way to improve your anaerobic endurance. They involve doing a series of exercises one after the other without resting or putting the bar down. My athletes usually do 6 reps per set of each exercise before immediately moving to the next exercise in the series. After completing all of the exercises, you will rest before repeating the complex. These are incredibly challenging, so choose a lighter weight than you might normally select. Remember: It's much less humiliating to start too light and have to add weight than it is to remove plates after you fail to get through the complex. The key is to perform each rep as fast as possible and move quickly from one exercise to the next. Below are three examples of complexes:

COMPLEX 1
Hang Snatch
Overhead Squat
Snatch Grip High Pull
Romanian Deadlift
Bent over Row
Deadlift
Rest 60 seconds, and repeat 6 times

COMPLEX 2
Front Raise
Reverse Curl
Hang Snatch
Hang Clean
Front Squat
Military Press
Good Morning
Back Squat
Rest 90 seconds, and repeat 5 times

COMPLEX 3

Overhead Triceps Extension

Back Squat

Good Morning

Push Press

Front Squat

Hang Clean

Romanian Deadlift

Bent over Row

Snatch

Overhead Squat

Rest 90 to 120 seconds, and repeat 4 or 5 times

Sean Sherk is known as one of the best-conditioned athletes in the world. On top of his grueling grappling and kickboxing practices, he also does stadium stair runs and conditioning circuits that include five 5-minute rounds in which he does one exercise for a minute and then another immediately following with no rest in between. He switches it up between tire flips, rope pulls, jumps, and other strongman or body weight-based exercises. It's no coincidence that he also is a world champion.

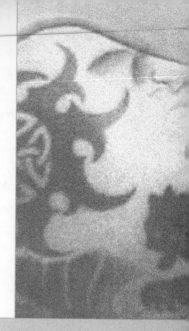

4 STRONGMAN TRAINING

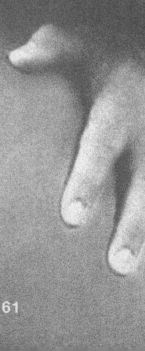

IF I HAD TO PICK JUST ONE METHOD OF TRAINING TO USE FOR the mixed martial artist, strongman training would be the weapon of choice. If you've ever caught part of the Met-Rx World's Strongest Man contest on ESPN, you're probably already familiar with strongman training. Performing exercises like tire flips, farmers walks, and keg presses is not only a fun way to break the monotony of conventional weight training; it's also an unbeatable method for developing true functional strength, speed, power, and endurance that will transfer directly to your performance in combat sports. All of my combat athletes and football players routinely compete in strongman challenges at my training facility, and they all say without question that it's their favorite day of every training week.

That said, strongman training requires some special equipment and space. Unless you happen to be the guy who races Grave Digger at monster truck rallies for a living, you probably don't have a four-hundred-pound rubber tire handy. You'll also need a big backyard or access to a spacious park or parking lot so you don't risk taking out a passing Boy Scout troop during your tire workouts. But believe me, the effort and expense you put into strongman training will come back to you tenfold when it's time to get it on on the mat or in the ring.

Below is a description of the best strongman training implements for combat athletes and their many uses.

Sandbags

Sandbags should be a staple in the training of any mixed martial artist. The beauty of sandbags is that unlike some of the other strongman training implements, they can be used almost anywhere (even in a stuffy public gym). Several companies sell sandbags with specially designed handles that are made just for training. See the Resources section at the back of the book for specific ordering information. If you don't want to buy a sandbag, you can make your own. Go to an Army Navy store and buy a sturdy medium-size duffel bag, then fill several plastic trash bags with sand and stuff them inside your duffel. The number of plastic bags you fill depends on how heavy you want to make the sandbag. Make sure to tightly seal both the inner bags and the outer bag before performing any exercises with the sandbag. If you don't want to deal with the hassle of the smaller plastic bags inside, you could add the sand directly to the duffel bag. The only problem is that this can get very messy and will make adjusting the weight of the bag more of a pain in the ass than it's worth. The ideal starting weight is highly individual, but most people usually will start with a 100-pound sandbag and adjust accordingly from there. You can increase or decrease the weight by adding or subtracting sand from the bag.

Sandbags challenge your strength, balance, stabilization, and coordination and provide an extremely brutal workout. When you lift a barbell, the weight is evenly distributed and never shifts. But when you lift a sandbag, the sand is constantly shifting around, which makes it incredibly challenging. In terms of combat sports, sandbag training is far more "sport specific" than standard weight lifting. Wrestling a sandbag from the floor up to your shoulder very closely approximates the kind of strength you will have to display in a fight. For example, in a judo throw, you need to move the weight of your opponent like you would a sandbag. When you're in a fight you have to move your own body plus your opponent's body weight. When you condition without additional resistance, it won't have as much of a carryover to the mat. Conditioning with extra resistance, such as sandbag training, has great carryover to the mat. Here are some of the best sandbag exercises:

Sandbag Clean from the Hang

Grab the sandbag on each end and bend over so the bag is just above your knees. Make sure your back is arched and your butt is out. Initiate the clean by explosively popping your hips forward and pulling the bag up to your upper chest. As it nears your chin, flip the bag over and throw your elbows forward to catch it. Reverse the motion and repeat.

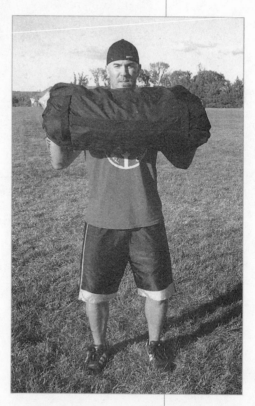

Sandbag Clean from the Floor

In this version, you start with the bag on the floor and squat down to grab it. Dead lift it off the ground in a deliberate, controlled motion, and once it clears your knees, finish it just like the Clean from the Hang.

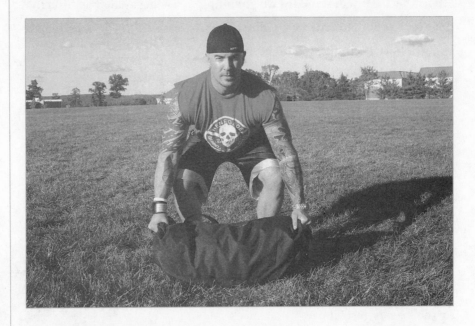

Sandbag Clean and Press from the Hang

After you have cleaned the bag up to your upper chest, use a slight knee bend and dip down to generate some momentum from your legs while simultaneously pushing the bag to lockout at arm's-length overhead.

Sandbag Clean and Press from the Floor

Clean the sandbag as you would in the Sandbag Clean from the Floor, and then press it from your shoulders to straight overhead.

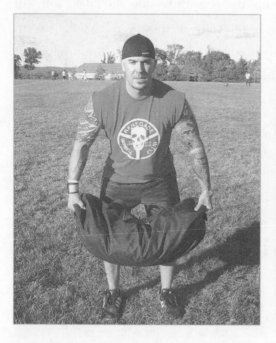 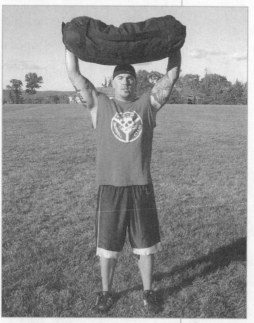

Sandbag Military Press

Simply clean the bag to your upper chest on the first rep and then perform standing overhead military presses. Do not put the bag down until you've completed the prescribed reps.

Sandbag Snatch

Start in the same position as the Sandbag Clean from the Hang and in one explosive motion lift the bag straight overhead to lockout at arm's length. This is done by initiating with an explosive popping forward of the hips while simultaneously pulling the bag straight up overhead.

Sandbag Shouldering

Straddle a sandbag. Then squat down over the bag and grab it underneath with both hands. Lift the bag up with one explosive motion by driving your hips forward and heaving the bag up to one shoulder. You will have to squat underneath the bag to catch it. Once you have the bag on your shoulder, stand up straight and steady yourself before dropping it back on the ground to start the next rep. Alternate shoulders throughout the set.

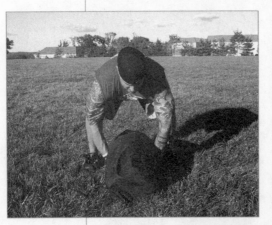

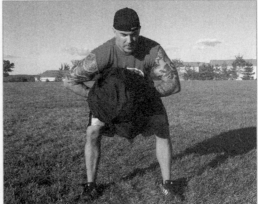

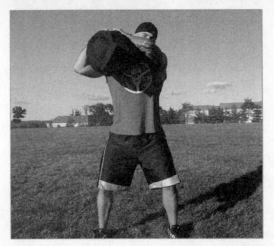

Sandbag Zercher Squat

Grab the bag with both arms underneath it like you would hold a baby. Then squat down below parallel while maintaining the arch in your back.

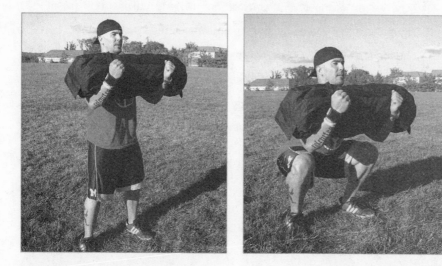

Sandbag Zercher Walk

Hold the bag just as you would in a Zercher Squat and walk for time or distance with it. This is great for conditioning and can be grueling.

Sandbag Rotational Throw

Hold the sandbag in the Sandbag Clean from the Hang position and twist to one side. Explosively rotate to the opposite side and throw the bag as far as you can. Quickly retrieve the bag and throw it in the opposite direction. Continue until finishing all of the prescribed reps.

Sandbag Bear Hug Walk

Simply bear hug the sandbag and walk with it for the prescribed amount of time or distance.

■ **How do I determine the weight of the object I am using for throwing exercises such as medicine-ball or sandbag throws?**

■ The weight of the object varies from athlete to athlete. The rule of thumb is that if you can throw the implement more than 100 feet, it is far too light to do anything to improve your speed; and conversely, if you can't throw it more than 10 feet, it is too heavy to use for speed development and actually becomes more of a strength exercise. Ideally, you want the medicine ball or sandbag you are using to fall somewhere in between that range; 30 to 60 feet is usually the optimal range for speed development in most individuals.

Kegs

One of the best and cheapest strongman implements is the beer keg. Some liquor stores will give you an old one, or you might have to give them a few bucks for it. The best scenario is to get a keg with a side tap so that you can add or subtract water as you wish. If that is not an option, try to get two or three kegs of different weights to use for different exercises. Like sandbags, kegs replicate the moving and ever-shifting weight of your opponent and are brutally hard and effective training implements. An empty keg is extremely light, so you usually will need to fill it at least halfway for it to be an effective training tool. For most keg training exercises, you will grab the keg on either end, holding it lengthwise in front of you. Below are some of the best keg training exercises (next to drinking, that is):

Keg Clean from the Hang

Grab the keg by the ends and hoist it to just above your knees while keeping your butt out, chest up, and back arched. Initiate the clean by explosively popping your hips forward and pulling the keg up to your upper chest. As you pull the keg up, dip under it slightly and catch it by throwing your elbows forward. Steady it in the rack position before reversing the motion and repeating.

Keg Clean from the Floor

Squat down and grab the keg at the ends with your arms completely straight and your back arched. With a controlled and deliberate motion, lift the keg until it clears your knees, then explosively drive your hips forward and clean the keg up to your shoulders.

Keg Clean and Press from the Hang

Once you clean the keg up to your upper chest and hold it at shoulder level, allow it to steady and let the water stop sloshing around for a second. Begin the pressing portion of the movement by using a slight knee dip to generate momentum and then explosively pressing the keg straight overhead to lockout at arm's length.

Keg Military Press

Clean the keg up to your upper chest and hold it at shoulder level on the first rep. After allowing the weight to stop sloshing around, press the weight straight overhead to lockout at arm's length. Lower the keg back to your chest and then press it back up again for the prescribed number of reps.

Keg Snatch from the Hang

Start with the keg just above your knees, your back arched and chest out. Initiate the movement by explosively driving your hips forward and locking out your knees while simultaneously pulling the keg straight up overhead to lockout in one swift motion.

Keg Snatch from the Floor

Squat down and grab the keg at the ends with your arms completely straight and your back arched. With a controlled and deliberate motion, lift the keg until it clears your knees; at that point explosively drive your hips forward, and in one swift motion pull the keg straight up overhead to lockout.

Overhead Keg Throw

Spread your legs wide enough to allow the keg to swing through them. Then grab the keg and stand up straight. Next, bend over with your back arched, chest up, and butt out, and start generating momentum by doing a few practice swings through your legs. When you decide you are ready to throw the keg, explosively pop your hips forward, lock your knees, and get up on your toes while launching the keg straight overhead and throwing it as far as you can. It is best to use a fairly light keg for this.

Sledgehammers

A sledgehammer is a great tool not only for conditioning but also for dramatically improving your grip strength, which is crucial for the combat athlete. Sledgehammers are readily found at well-equipped hardware stores, and these exercises don't require as much space as the sandbag or the keg. While there are lots of ways to use a sledgehammer, I prefer to use it primarily for swings. The two swings described here are the ones I use with my combat athletes, and we primarily use an 8- or 10-pound sledgehammer.

Cross-Body Sledgehammer Swing

For this exercise you'll need a rubber tire or a sandbag in addition to your sledgehammer. Start by placing the rubber tire or sandbag in front of your left foot. Then grab the sledgehammer in your right hand, bring it up over your right shoulder, and swing down at the tire or sandbag. Complete all repetitions on one side before switching to the other side.

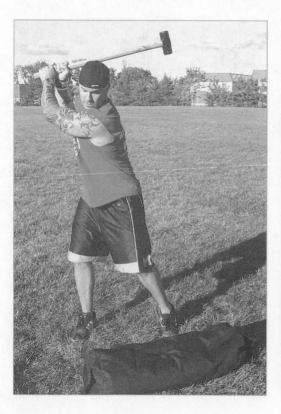 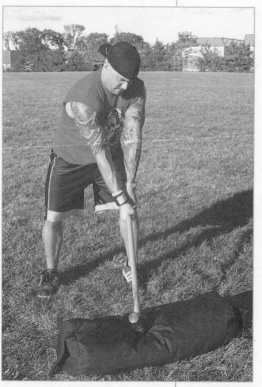

Overhead Sledgehammer Swing

Place the rubber tire or sandbag in front of you. Using both hands, bring the sledgehammer directly over your head and swing straight down to the tire or sandbag. Make sure to brace your abs tightly as you perform this exercise.

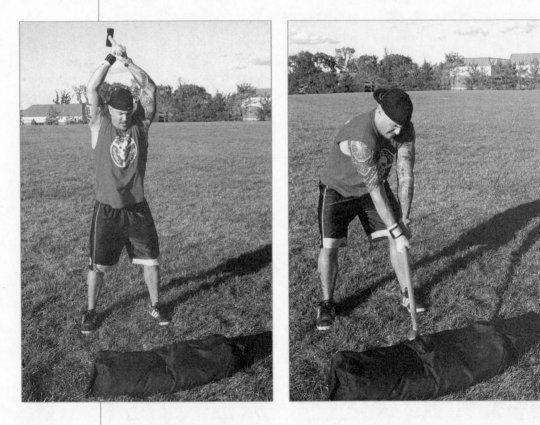

Dragging Sleds

A weighted dragging sled is one of the most versatile and effective training tools for combat conditioning. It works both your upper and lower body, and you can change your routine depending upon your training goals. Athletes usually use the dragging sled in a yard or open field. The sleds are designed so you can add weight to them, adding to their versa-tility. The overall goal is to drag the sled for a prescribed distance, amount of time, or both. If you are training for speed, you'll want to keep the weight of the sled fairly light and keep the times and distances short. If you are training for strength or a combination of speed and strength, you will want to use moderate to heavy weight over short to moderate distances. If you are training for strength and endurance conditioning, you will want to use light, moderate, or heavy weights and drag for 60 seconds and longer.

These are the sled-dragging methods I use with my combat athletes:

Forward Sled Drag

This can be done by holding two separate handles attached to the sled, either out in front of you in press position or directly behind you. Another option is to attach the sled to a weight-lifting belt around your waist.

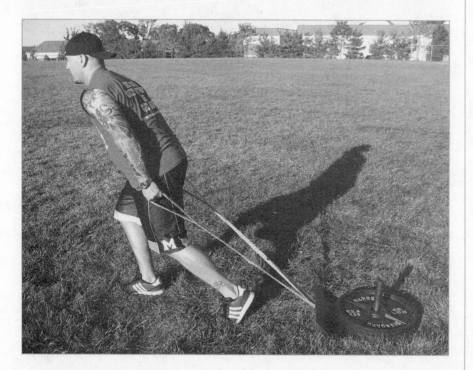

Backward Sled Drag

This is a great movement to build up strength and endurance in your quadriceps. Drag the sled backward by either holding the handles at arm's length in front of you or by attaching the strap to a belt.

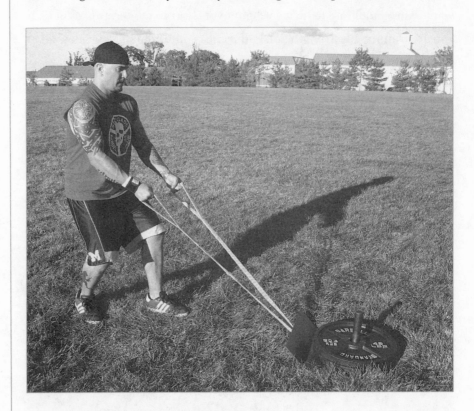

Sled Chest Press

For this exercise you will need a pair of blast straps, which can be purchased at EliteFTS.com or elsewhere. Blast straps are long straps with single D handle attachments on one end. The other end has an open loop with a carabiner that can be attached to anything. Attach the blast straps to the sled and press forward as you walk. Make sure to time it just right so that you press and then rapidly walk forward during the eccentric/negative portion of the press in order to maintain tension throughout. Continue walking throughout the set until you have reached the distance you set out to reach or you have completed all the prescribed reps.

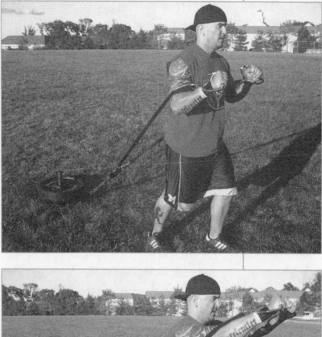

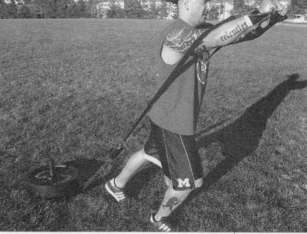

Sled Row

Attach two single straps with handles to the sled and begin walking backward as you row the sled in toward you. Continue walking and rowing until you have reached the prescribed distance or number of reps.

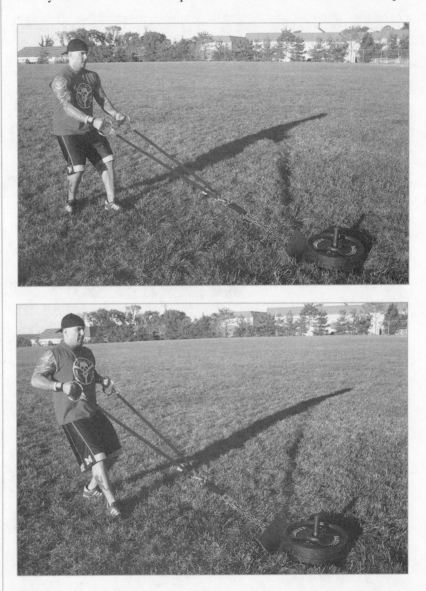

Sled Rope Row

Attach the sled to a thick-diameter (2.5- to 3-inch) rope that is at least 50 feet long, and grab the other end. Using a hand-over-hand rowing motion, pull the sled toward you. If you do this with light weights, you can row the sled all the way in and then grab the end and sprint until the rope is straightened again, and once again row it all the way in. Depending on the length of the rope and how long it takes you to row it in, repeat this for 2 to 5 reps.

Another option is to load the sled with heavy weight that will take you 30 to 60 seconds to row all the way in and do just one brutal set.

In my opinion, the best sleds are available at EliteFTS.com. If you do not want to purchase a sled, you can make your own using a heavy tire and a rope. The tire should be roughly 40 to 50 pounds. If you cannot find a tire that weighs this much, you can try adding cement to an old car tire.

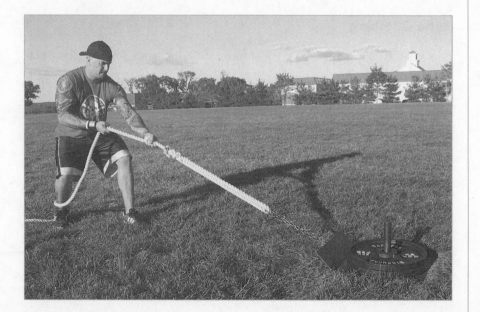

Thick-Diameter Ropes

Thick ropes (2.5 to 3 inches in diameter) are great for a variety of pulling exercises. You'll want a rope that is at least 50 feet long if possible. Pulling strength is very important for the mixed martial artist, as is grip strength. The great thing about the thick ropes is that they work both qualities while also incorporating your core and improving rotational strength. The three best rope exercises follow:

Rope Rows

As described in the sled training section (page 77). You also can attach a thick rope to a car or truck. Find an open parking lot or quiet side street and have a friend behind the wheel of the vehicle to keep the wheels straight. Put the car in neutral and turn off the engine. Attach the rope to the front bumper or grill and stand back 50 feet. Now you can begin pulling the rope toward you, dragging the vehicle.

Rope Climbing

This is pretty self-explanatory—just hang the rope from a high ceiling and climb like you used to do in high school gym class. You can also climb two ropes by holding one with each hand. This two-rope version is for stronger, more-advanced athletes.

Tug-of-War

This is also just like high school gym class but is an incredible full-body exercise for the combat athlete. Tug-of-war can be done with a partner or in teams. It's a great exercise for building up strength and endurance throughout the entire body, and it simulates combat in that you often

- **We all know that grip training is very important for MMA competitors. What are some of the best grip-training exercises or techniques?**

- Some of my favorite grip exercises are:

Any exercise performed with the fat bar, including:

- Fat Bar Hold
- Fat Bar Chin-up
- Fat Bar Chin-up Hang

Other great grip exercises:

- Towel Chin-up
- Towel Hang
- Hexagon Dumbbell Hold
- Farmers Walk
- Rope Row with 2.5- to 3-inch-diameter rope
- Tug-of-War with 2.5- to 3-inch-diameter rope
- Keg Lifts

will be in an intense isometric contraction without moving for several seconds at a time while contracting maximally. Tug-of-war exercises will do wonders for your grip strength as well. This is a great exercise to finish a normal workout or strongman day, as the challenge of competition can bring out the best in you and allow you to end your workout on a high note.

Tire Flip

Nothing beats the tire flip, especially for the combat athlete. It's a fantastic total body exercise, working just about every muscle in your body. This exercise also develops unbelievable real-world strength and power, not to mention incredible levels of conditioning. The only requirement is a big tractor tire, preferably in the neighborhood of 350 to 500 pounds. Look for a junkyard that has old tires—you usually can get one for free. Another option is to contact a construction company and ask if they have any tractor tires they are no longer using.

To properly execute a tire flip, squat all the way down and get your hands underneath the tire while keeping your back arched. Your chest should be touching the tire and you should be on the balls of your feet, leaning into the tire slightly. As you lift the tire, explode forward while driving your chest into it. When it clears your knees, quickly transition your hands from the underneath lifting position to a pressing position and explosively push the tire to complete the flip. Repeat for the prescribed number of reps.

This exercise develops explosive power, brute strength, and incredible endurance all in one set. To get the tire moving, you need to have a very powerful posterior chain, which is of critical importance to the mixed martial artist. To even move the tire in the first place, you need explosive power, which also comes into play when you transition from the lifting to the pushing phase. And a set of 5 to 8 tire flips will do more for your conditioning than just about anything else. In fact, I've found that after a set of tire flips, it's usually impossible to get up off the ground for at least a minute.

Farmers Walk

The farmers walk can be done with dumbbells or specially designed farmers walk handles (see the Resources section in the back of the book). Basically, all you are doing is picking up the implements and carrying them for a prescribed time or distance. Use the heaviest weight you can handle—this builds great strength and endurance throughout the entire body and works the traps and grip musculature especially hard. Another benefit of the farmers walk is that it greatly increases stability of the core along with the hip, knee, and ankle joints. Farmers walks are great to use as a finisher to your normal workout. For this purpose, two sets of fifty yards with the heaviest weight you can handle works perfectly.

The Prowler

The Prowler is a heavy metal pushing and dragging implement. It is basically a sled on skis with two upright poles that you can grab onto and push or drag backward. If you had to pick one, the Prowler is a better option than a sled because it can be pushed as well as pulled. To push it, hold onto the upright handles or grab the low attachment and push from there. Either way, this is a killer conditioning exercise for combat athletes.

Further away from a fight for MMA, we will use strongman-only days as a combo type strength and strength and endurance day. But as competition nears, these days are strictly geared at improving conditioning. If you choose to add some strongman work to the end of your regular weight-training workouts, strictly for conditioning purposes I recommend picking one exercise performed with a sledgehammer, keg, or sandbag and doing timed rounds of work. For example, you could swing a sledgehammer at a truck tire or a sandbag for timed 30- to 60-second rounds, followed by a 1-minute rest period. Over time the goal is to increase the time under tension while maintaining the same rest period. Another great option is to do hang cleans or hang clean and presses with a keg or sandbag for similarly timed rounds and rest intervals. One of the best strongman finishers for the combat athlete is to perform tire flips with a 300 to 500-pound tractor trailer tire. You could try to perform as many reps as possible in a 30- to 60-second period followed by a 90- to 180-second rest interval.

However you choose to implement strongman training into your program is up to you. What matters more than anything else is that you do it. There is no more effective method of training for the combat athlete, and the exercises included in this chapter need to be in the arsenal of every serious mixed martial artist.

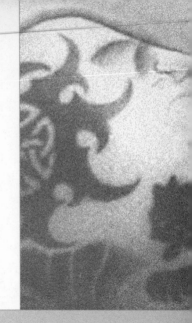

5   KICK-ASS SPEED AND STRENGTH

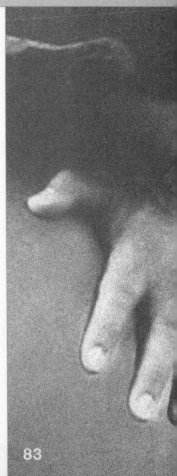

As I mentioned earlier, Matt Hughes is known as one of the strongest guys in his weight class. When he fought the legendary Royce Gracie, it was one of the most anticipated fights of all time. The match was scheduled for three five-minute rounds, and the crowd was split down the middle. The first time they tied up against the cage, Hughes picked up Gracie and dropped him on the ground. At that point, all of Gracie's skill was not enough to combat Hughes's incredible strength. They were on the ground, which is Gracie's domain, where no one wants to be with him. Hughes's strength was so great that he was able to muscle Gracie into a kimora. When Gracie wouldn't tap out, Hughes finally released the hold and then overpowered Gracie into a side mount, at which point Gracie gave him his back. Matt finally rained down punches on the back of Gracie's head, and the ref was left with no choice but to stop the fight. Gracie may have been the more skilled fighter, but Hughes's strength was just too great for him, and he was out-matched. Hughes's strength won the fight.

If you watch any successful mixed martial artist, you will notice that he almost always possesses above-average levels of both speed and strength. Without these two qualities, your chances of victory are severely compromised. You need speed to deliver blinding punches and kicks as well as to shoot in for or avoid takedowns. You need strength to get out of sticky situations or manhandle your opponent into the positions you want him to be in. Strength also can often negate good technique, as I described with Hughes's win over Gracie. One is not more important than the other, but the combination is lethal—and essential. If your opponent possesses both and you do not, you may be in for a world of hurt.

I'm addressing training methods for speed and strength together because they are inseparable. To get faster you usually have to get stronger, and to break through strength plateaus you usually have to get faster. There are three ways to induce maximal muscular tension, which is what you need to get stronger, faster, and more muscular. The first of these is the maximal-effort method. This involves lifting a heavy weight, usually above 90 percent of your 1 rep max (the most weight you can lift for one repetition on a particular exercise, abbreviated 1RM) for 1 to 3 reps. This is the best way to get stronger fast. When you lift a really heavy weight, your nervous system is forced to recruit more muscle fibers. That allows for more muscle growth (that is, if you're eating enough) and improved coordination of the muscles involved.

The second method is known as the repeated-effort method. This is a bodybuilding technique that most guys use when they first start lifting (whether they know it or not). It involves using moderately heavy weights and doing multiple sets of 8 to 12 reps to the point of muscular failure. For reasons I'll explain later, I do not advise training to failure—in fact, I actively discourage it.

The third method, which I prefer, is the modified-repeated effort method, in which you perform a set until you're 1 to 2 reps shy of failure. This is the safest way to reap the muscle-building benefits of the

---

TIPS FROM THE CAGE

■ **Is isometric work of any benefit to the combat athlete?**

■ Yes. Many of the contractions in a wrestling match or fight are isometric in nature. You need to be able to hold onto certain positions for an extended period of time. You will often see two combat athletes locked together on the mat, both of them fiercely holding an isometric contraction. Slowly but surely the one with greater endurance will end up with the upper hand. Isometric work can be done in your endurance workouts for timed holds, or you can incorporate isometric work into your weight-training workouts. One good way of mixing isometric work into your conditioning workouts is to simply bear hug a punching bag with your arms and legs wrapped around it and hang for as long as you can. Another option is to just lie on the floor with the bag and simply squeeze it with both your arms and legs for 15 to 45 seconds. On strength-training days you could mix your isometrics right into a normal set. For example, on a set of chin-ups, hold a certain position for 15 to 30 seconds at the end of the set. Another option is to do a brief isometric contraction on each rep. For example, stop at the halfway point of each rep and pause for 6 seconds before completing the rep and returning to the dead hang position. Do this for 5 to 10 reps per set.

---

repeated-effort method while minimizing the risk of injury or overtraining. The goal with this method is to recruit a large number of muscle fibers and thoroughly work them to fatigue—not absolute failure—which in turn stimulates growth.

I've already covered many of the greatest strength-building exercises in the strongman section. In this section, I'll go over the more traditional and most effective strength-building exercises.

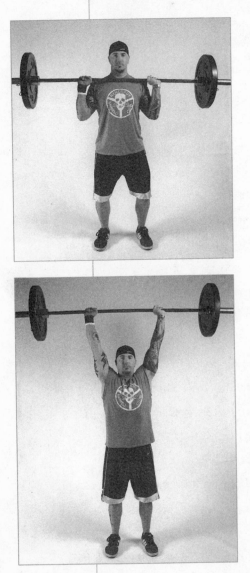

Standing Military Press

The shoulders are crucially important muscles for combat, and they also are very injury prone. The standing military press is the best shoulder exercise there is and will help prevent injuries to this area.

Begin by setting the bar in a rack at upper chest height. Grab the bar with an overhand, shoulder-width grip, and nudge it off the rack so that you now support it at shoulder height with your arms. Squeeze the bar as tight as you can and press it straight up overhead. You need to press in a bit of an arc to get it around your head. You'll also need to move your head back out of the way and then move it back forward to lock out the weight. Make sure to keep your back arched and do not lean too far backward. If you find yourself leaning too far, reduce the weight.

Push Press

This is performed exactly like a military press, except that before you press the weight up overhead you dip down into a quarter-squat position and use a strong leg drive to assist you in pressing the weight up. As soon as you start driving with your legs, start pressing. Do all these things simultaneously to get the most from your leg drive. Lower the weight to your chest before dipping down into a quarter-squat position for the next rep.

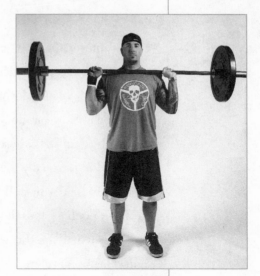

Standing Dumbbell Press

Hold dumbbells at shoulder level and press overhead. Dumbbells allow you to get a slightly greater range of motion than a barbell can offer, and they work more of the stabilizer muscles (including those of the core).

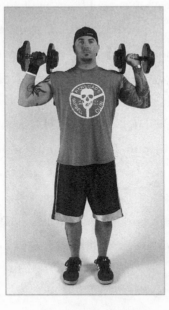
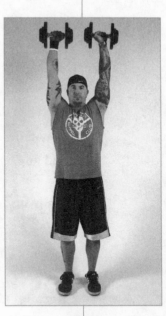

Pull-up

This is one of the best exercises to stimulate strength gains in the lats, upper back, biceps, brachialis, and forearms. One need look no further than the body of elite-level male gymnasts to see what a steady diet of pull-ups and chin-ups can do for your physique. But for the combat athlete (as well as the gymnast), these muscles are for more than just show. All these muscles, but especially the lats and upper back, help you deliver powerful strikes and help you pull your opponent in the direction you want him. Strong upper back muscles also act as decelerators, which keep your shoulders safe. When you throw a punch, the muscles of the upper back are responsible for decelerating your arm safely and keeping your shoulders intact. Without a strong upper back you will be at greater risk for injury.

Grab the bar with your palms facing away from you and a shoulder-width grip. Drop to a dead hang, with your arms completely straight. Pull up until your chest hits the bar, while fully contracting your shoulder blades and squeezing your lats at the top. Lower yourself with control and allow your arms to completely straighten before beginning the next rep.

When doing any form of pull-up or chin-up, try to think of your arms as nothing more than hooks, and concentrate on pulling with your lats and forcing them to do the majority of the work.

Chin-up

This is basically a pull-up with your palms facing you instead of away from you. This exercise hits the biceps in addition to the lats.

Parallel Chin-up

This is performed exactly the same way as a regular chin-up. The only difference is that your palms are facing each other. These can be done on a specifically designed apparatus that has two parallel handles sticking out of the middle of a normal-chin up bar, or by hanging a parallel grip pull-down handle over a chin-up bar. As with all forms of chin-ups, make sure to extend your arms completely at the bottom and pull until your chest hits the bar with your shoulder blades fully retracted at the top.

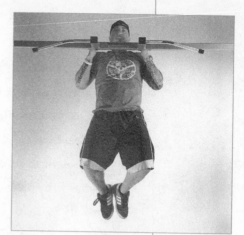

Towel Chin-up

This is a great version of chin-ups for the combat athlete, because not only does it train the all-important lats and upper back, but it also greatly overloads the grip muscles. Loop a thick towel over a chin-up bar and grab an end of it in each hand. Now perform a chin-up as normal. You'll really need to squeeze the ends of the towel to hold on.

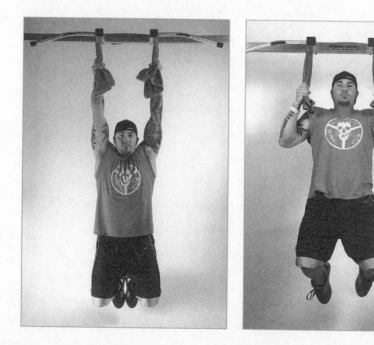

Face Pull

This is an outstanding upper back exercise and is performed by attaching the rope handle to the top pulley of a cable station. While standing perfectly upright, extend your arms straight out in front of you and grab the handles. Step back a foot or so until you feel tension on the cable. Row the weight toward your face and pull your elbows back as far behind you as you can. Make sure to fully retract your shoulder blades and pause briefly in the retracted position. This strengthens the muscles of the upper back and rotator cuff musculature, which is very important for preventing common injuries in combat sports.

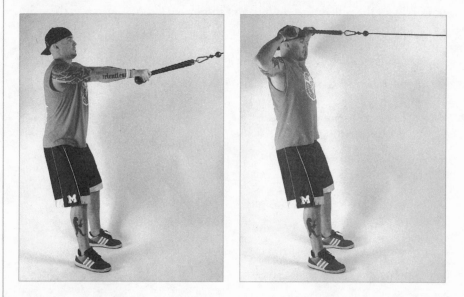

Incline Y Raise

Lie facedown on a 45-degree incline bench with dumbbells in each hand. With your arms straight, lift the dumbbells as high as you can while keeping them straight out in front of you. Hold the top position for a second before lowering.

Blast Strap Inverted Rows

For this exercise, you can either use blast straps or gymnastics rings. (Similar to rings, blast straps are nylon tethers with adjustable metal handles that can be used to perform a number of intense body-weight exercises. You can find them on EliteFTS.com.) Loop the blast straps or gymnastics rings around the top of a power rack and set the handles about 2½ feet off the ground. Lie down on your back on the floor beneath the handles, reach up, and grab them. Raise your body off the floor, straighten your hips, and lock your knees while hanging from the handles. Now simply row your body straight up, making sure to pull your shoulder blades all the way back at the top.

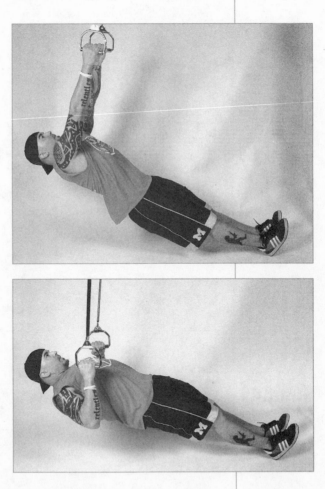

Not only does this movement work your upper back and lats, but it also forces you to stabilize throughout your core because your body is moving, as opposed to just your limbs. This makes this exercise a superior rowing movement for combat athletes. To increase the difficulty, you can wear a weighted vest.

One-Arm Dumbbell Row

You'll need a bench or other stationary object for this exercise. Pick up a dumbbell with one hand and place your opposite hand on the bench to support your body weight. Keeping your back arched, allow your lats to stretch fully in the start position. Initiate the movement by pulling with the lats and row the weight up until the dumbbell touches the side of your torso.

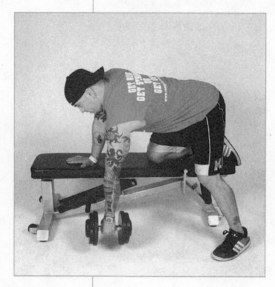
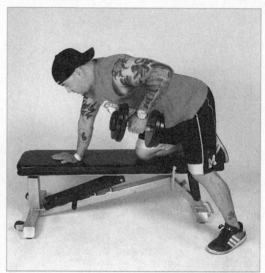

Bent-over Barbell Row

Grab a barbell with an overhand grip and stand straight up. With your chest out and shoulder blades back, descend nearly into the bottom position of a Romanian dead lift. From this position, row the bar up to your midsection while contracting your shoulder blades at the top. This is a great exercise for building strength in the upper back.

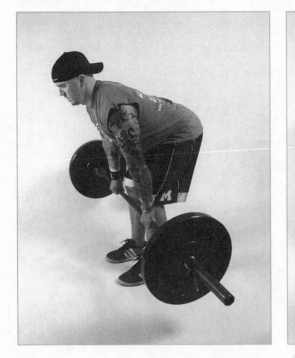
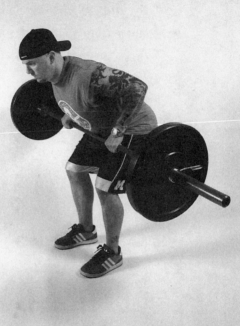

Bent-over Reverse Grip Barbell Row

This is done exactly like the barbell row, except that you grab the bar with your palms facing up.

High Pull

Stand with a shoulder-width grip on the bar, palms facing down, and bend over until it is just above your knees. While keeping your back arched and chest up, explosively straighten your body by driving your hips forward and getting up on your toes. As you straighten out, pull the bar up to mid-chest height, being sure to initiate the pull with a shrugging motion.

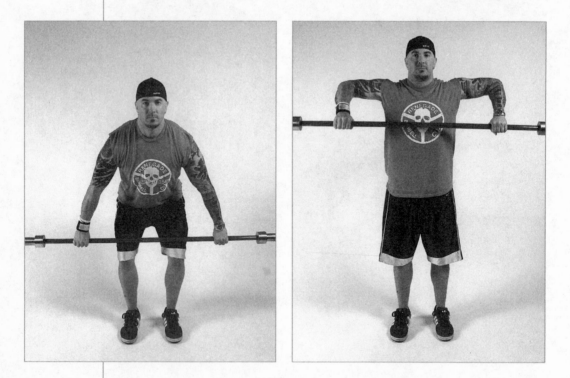

Standing Barbell Triceps Extension

Grab the bar with a shoulder-width or slightly closer grip, palms facing away from you, and hold it at arm's length, directly overhead. Hinge at the elbows, allowing only your forearms to move, and lower the weight straight down behind your head. Get a full stretch in the triceps before pushing the weight back up to lockout.

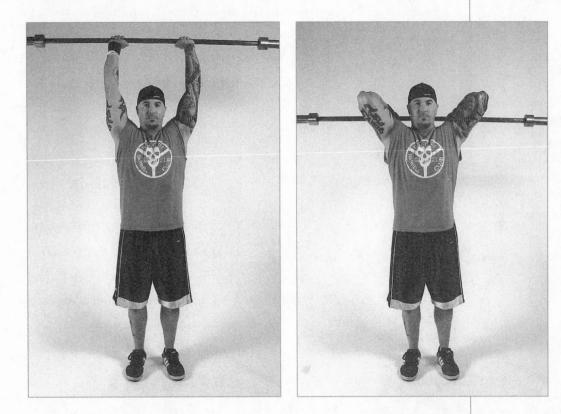

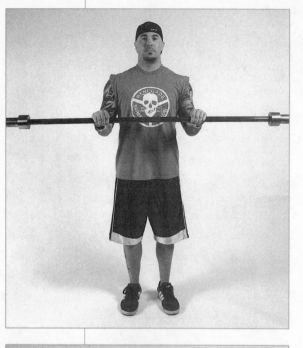

Reverse Curl

Stand up straight and grab the bar with a shoulder-width grip and your palms facing down. Hinge at the elbows, allowing only your forearms to move, and curl the bar up as far as you can without bringing your elbows forward or bending your wrists.

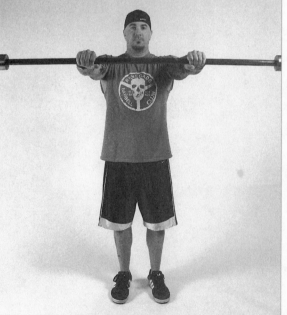

Front Raise

Grab the bar with a shoulder-width overhand grip while standing straight up. Bend your elbows slightly and keep them in that position. Now simply raise the bar until your arms are parallel with the ground. Lower with control and repeat.

Punch Press

This movement trains the serratus anterior, the muscle below your pecs that typically is only visible when you raise your hands overhead. The serratus holds the shoulder blades to the rib cage, making it a crucial muscle for shoulder health and a major source of punching power. Lie down on a bench with a dumbbell in one hand and the other on your stomach. Press the dumbbell straight overhead to lockout. From there, let your shoulder drop as low as you can on the side of the bench, and then reverse the motion by reaching up as high as you can while keeping your arm locked out. Do all the prescribed reps with one arm, then switch arms.

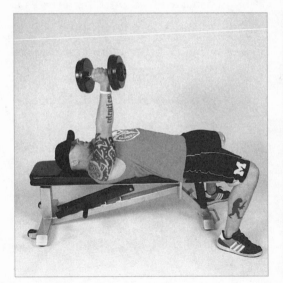 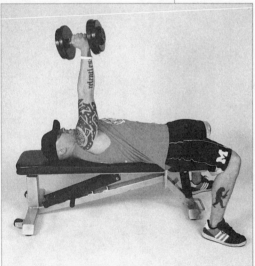

Flat Dumbbell Press

Grab two dumbbells and lie down on a flat bench. Keep your shoulder blades back and your elbows tucked with your palms facing in. Press the weights up in a straight line and then lower with control. Make sure to squeeze the dumbbells as tightly as possible throughout the set. This, along with the Incline Dumbbell Press (page 99) and one-arm versions, develops the muscles of the chest, shoulders, and triceps. For combat athletes, dumbbells always should be used in place of barbells for the majority of pressing exercises. This is to minimize the risk of injury when lifting extremely heavy weights, and it also increases stability in the joints.

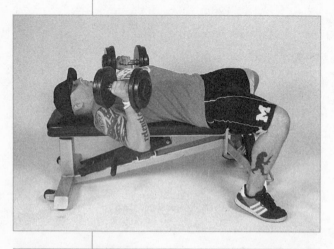

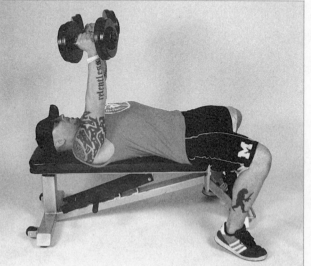

Incline Dumbbell Press

This is the same as a flat dumbbell press, except that it is performed on an incline bench set between 30 and 40 degrees.

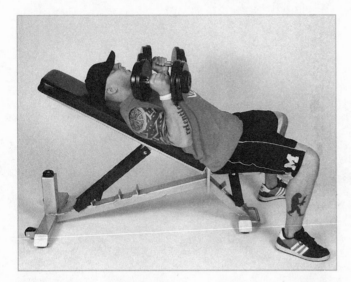

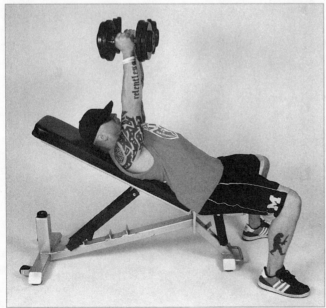

One-Arm Flat Dumbbell Press. Perform this just as you would the flat dumbbell press, only using one dumbbell and working one side at a time while keeping the hand of the nonworking arm on your stomach. You'll have to keep your abs braced to fight your body's tendency to rotate toward the side that's weighted.

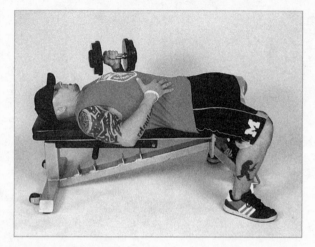

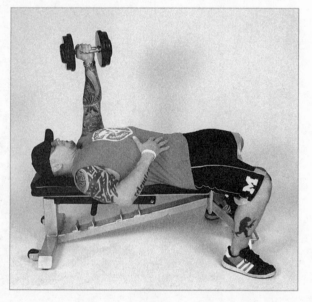

One-Arm Incline Dumbbell Press. Perform this as you would the Incline Dumbbell Press, but use only one arm.

Chain Suspended/Blast Strap Push-up

You'll need either blast straps, gymnastic rings, or two lengths of chain (from a hardware store) for this exercise. Set a bar high in a power rack. Loop two same-length chains, rings, or blast straps around the bar so that they hang down a few feet off the floor. (If you're using chains, wrap a towel around them for hand padding.) From there, grab the chains or handles and put your feet up on a bench so that your body is suspended in the air. Perform push-ups as normal, being sure to keep your entire body tight throughout the exercise.

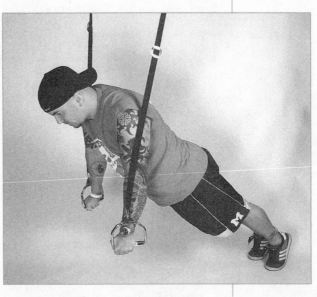

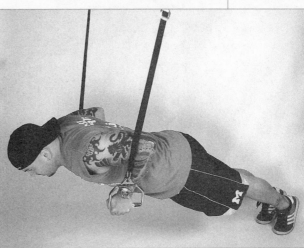

One-Arm Standing Cable Press

Attach a single D handle to an adjustable cable stack and set the height of the cable slightly below shoulder level. If you are holding the handle with your left hand, your right leg should be out in front of you with your left leg back (just as if you were going to throw a punch with your left arm). Press straight ahead explosively while rotating at the hips. This is a great exercise for improving punching power, and it strengthens not only the chest, shoulders, and triceps, but the core as well.

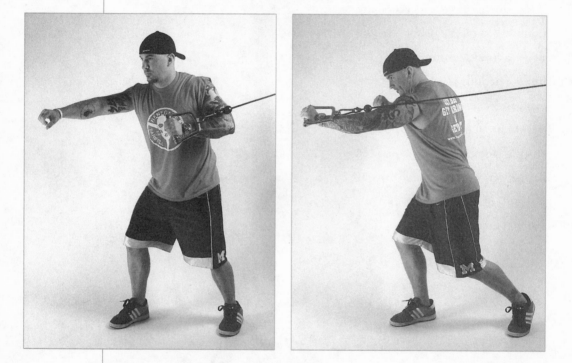

Plank

When it comes to training the abdominals and core, it pays to focus on developing the ability to resist movement. When your opponent is trying to move you one way and you are trying to stay put, your abs need to contract intensely to prevent movement.

The plank, or abdominal bridge, is one of the best exercises for building this type of strength. To perform this exercise, get down into a push-up position and rest your weight on your forearms. The goal is to hold this position with your abs tightly contracted and back arched properly for 1 to 3 minutes. Once you've mastered 3 minutes, you can increase the difficulty of the exercise by having someone place a weight on your back or by wearing a weighted vest.

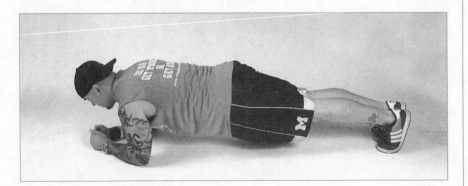

Side Plank

This exercise targets the obliques while providing the same benefits as the regular version of the plank. Lie down on your right side and support your weight on your right forearm, your legs extended with your left

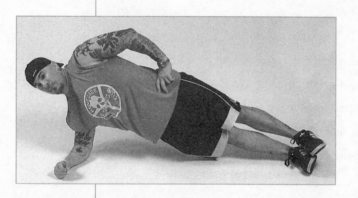

leg resting on your right so your body forms a straight line. Place your left hand on your left hip. Your weight is now being supported by your forearm and the outside of your right foot. Hold this position for up to 3 minutes, then switch sides.

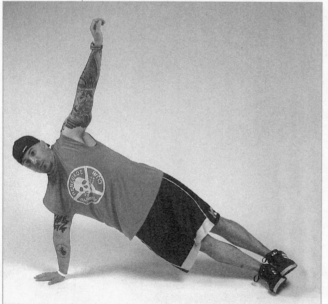

Advanced Side Plank

To increase the difficulty of this exercise, straighten both the support arm and non-working arm to form a T with your upper body. When this version gets easier, hold a weight in the arm that is up in the air.

Barbell Russian Twist

This is a great exercise for developing rotational strength, which is critically important to the combat athlete. Stick the end of a barbell in a corner (or create a corner with two boxes or other objects) and pad the wall with a towel to prevent damage. Grab the other end of the bar with both arms extended out in front of you. Initiate the movement by lowering the barbell down to one side until it is at hip level. Reverse the movement with an explosive contraction of the obliques by rotating back up to the start position while keeping both arms locked. Pause at the start position for a second and then lower the bar to the opposite side.

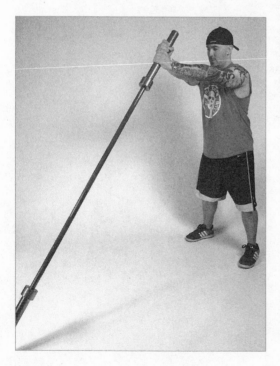
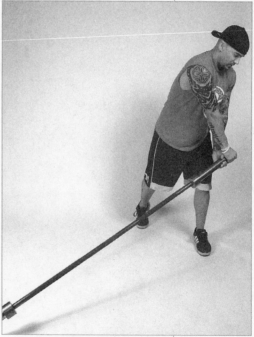

Cable Woodchopper

Attach a single D handle to a cable stack and set it slightly below shoulder height. Grab the handle with both hands and stand with your right side to the cable stack, about three feet from the machine. Extend your arms straight out in front of you, then brace your core and explosively rotate to the opposite side with a powerful contraction of the obliques. Return to the start position with control before performing the next rep. Finish all reps, then switch sides. This is another great exercise for developing the all-important rotational strength that every combat athlete needs.

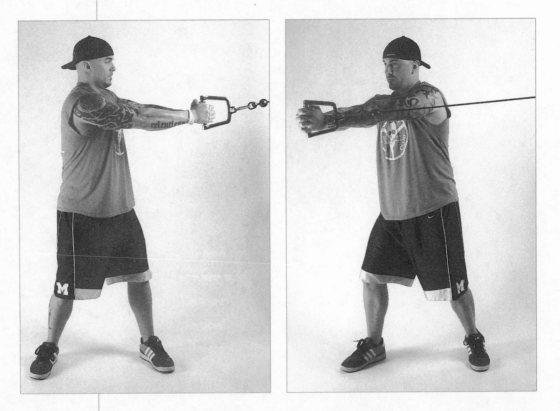

Hanging Knee Raise

Grab a chin-up bar with your palms facing away from you and hang with your arms straight. Bend your legs and bring them up so that they are parallel with the floor (or slightly below). That is the start position for every rep. By contracting your abs, lift your legs as high as you can so that they hit your chest and your pelvis rounds under you. To increase the difficulty of this exercise, straighten your legs at the start of each rep.

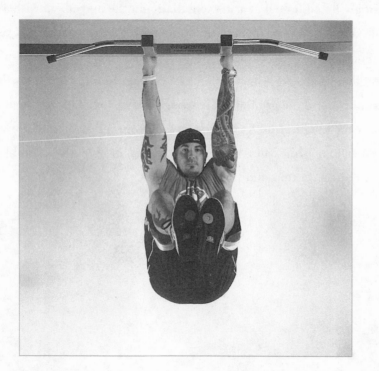

Modified Turkish Get-up

This is a great "total body ab exercise" for the combat athlete, as you find yourself flat on your back struggling against resistance to get to your feet just like you would in the cage. Grab a dumbbell and place it within reach. Lie down on the ground with your right knee bent and right foot flat on the ground. Your left leg should be straight and your left arm should be straight out to your side at a 45-degree angle. Using your right hand, grab a dumbbell and hold it at arm's length. Begin the movement with a powerful contraction of your abs while attempting to sit up. As you rise off the floor, make sure to keep your right arm perpendicular with the ground and pointing straight up at the ceiling. Roll to your left side and lift your butt off the ground while straightening your hips. In the top position your weight should be supported by your left hand and the side of your left foot while your right arm remains straight with dumbbell in hand. Repeat all reps and then switch sides.

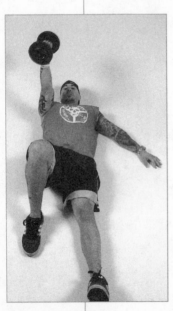
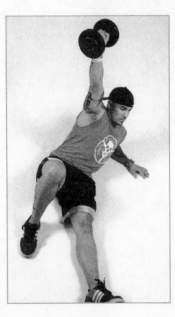
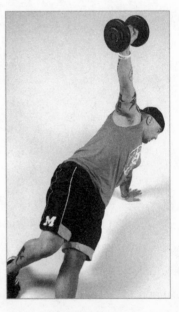

Decline Sit-up

You'll need a partner for this exercise. Set a bench at a 30- to 45-degree decline by propping one end up on a box. Bend your legs and keep your feet flat on the box while your partner holds your feet. Allow your head to hang off the end of the bench so that you can hold a dumbbell behind your head without it hitting the bench. Initiate the movement by contracting your abs, and then perform a sit-up as you normally would, only coming up to the point where the tension is about to be released from your abs, about three quarters of the way up.

Dumbbell Hand Walk

Hold a pair of dumbbells and get on the floor in push-up position, supporting yourself on the weights. Now reach your left arm forward and plant it on the floor a few inches in front of you, as if you had taken a step forward with your hand. Do the same with the right hand, so that both hands line up with each other again. Now, keeping your knees straight, use your ankles to walk your feet forward so that your arms are directly under you again—you will end up in the same push-up position you started in, but you'll be a few inches forward. That's 1 rep. Continue to do this for the prescribed reps or distance. Make sure to maintain proper posture without allowing your hips to sag too low. Keep your abs tightly braced throughout the exercise.

Alligator Walk

You will need a 25- or 45-pound weight plate with a decent-sized lip and a floor on which the plate can slide easily (a waxed floor would work well, which you can avoid scratching by wrapping the plate in a towel). Get down in push-up position and hook the toes of both feet onto the lip of the plate. Walk just as you did in the Dumbbell Hand Walk, while keeping your legs straight and abs tight.

Squat

Squats are one of the greatest total-body exercises you can do and simply the best leg exercise there is. Leg strength is of the utmost importance to combat athletes, because that is where all your power generates from. Without strong legs you never will be able to deliver powerful strikes or withstand the onslaught of your opponents.

Begin the exercise by getting into the proper setup. Before unracking the bar, make sure to take an even grip and squeeze your shoulder blades together. To create a bigger shelf to rest the bar, grip as comfortably close as possible; this will be anywhere from 4 to 12 inches outside of your shoulders. Rest the bar on your traps, not on your neck, and be sure to squeeze it as hard as you can.

Take a slightly wider than shoulder-width stance and point your toes out slightly. Keeping your chest high and your head up, inhale deeply

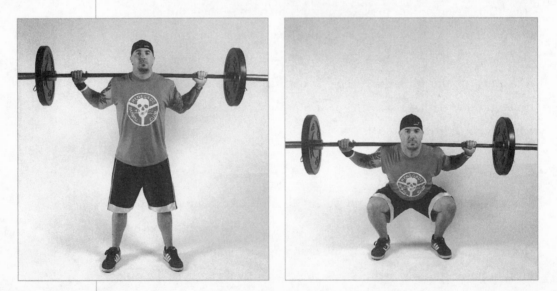

and fill your abdomen with air. This is a key point and must be practiced. You do not want to breathe in through your chest and allow your shoulders to rise. As you fill your belly with air, your abs will push out against your waistband as you descend. Start the descent by breaking at the hips and sitting back and down. Squat all the way down to below parallel, making sure to keep your back tightly arched (refrain from looking down). Once you have hit rock bottom, exhale and explode back to the top.

Front Squat

Set a loaded bar in a power rack at upper-chest height. Grab the bar with a shoulder-width grip and throw your elbows all the way forward as far as possible. Allow your wrists to bend back and rest the bar on your upper chest right below your throat. Keep your elbows pointing forward throughout the lift and don't let them drop toward the floor.

The execution is exactly the same as a regular squat. Break at the hips and push your glutes back while sitting back and down. Descend until your thighs are parallel with the ground and then explosively drive back up to the start position.

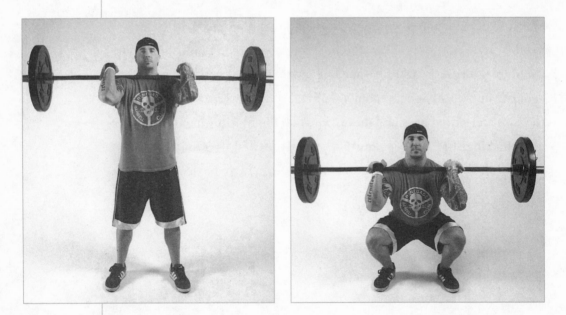

Box Squat

The box squat is the best exercise there is for strengthening the hip musculature. The hips are your body's center of power. When delivering a blow, power originates in the lower body and is transferred up through the hips to the core and upper body.

Load a barbell and then place a box that's a little below knee height a few inches behind you. When you squat, your butt will touch the box and your thighs will be parallel to the floor. Take a wider stance than you would for regular squats, positioning your feet about one and a half times shoulder width. Squat down, focusing on staying upright (think of lowering yourself into a chair). When you sit down on the box, your shins should be nearly perpendicular to the floor and your entire body should be tight. After a slight pause, explode back up by driving your traps back into the bar and pushing out on the sides of your feet, simultaneously driving your hips forward.

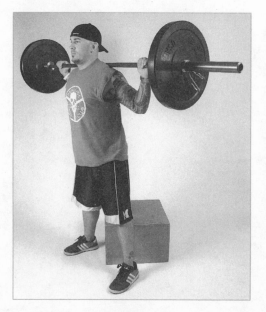
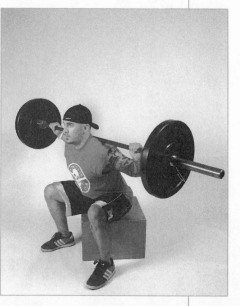

Belt Squat

This is another exercise that ideally requires a special machine to perform it optimally. A belt squat machine is a platform with a cable attachment in the middle of it. To perform the belt squat, you attach a specially designed belt to the cable and stand on the platform directly over it. The cable loops under the back of the machine and attaches to a weight stack, which provides the extra resistance when you squat. However, if you don't have access to a belt squat machine, you could get a belt squat belt and attach weights to it and squat while standing on top of two boxes. This is a great exercise for people with back problems that prevent them from squatting. Just about everyone can belt squat with no problems whatsoever. This form of squat works well for high-rep squatting because the lower back is not loaded at all. The lack of lower-back loading makes belt squats one of my favorite and most frequently prescribed exercises.

Zercher Squat

Hold the bar in the crook of your elbows and squat as usual. This will pull you forward, so you have to fight to stay upright. For combat athletes this exercise not only builds great core strength and stability but mental and physical toughness as well. It is very difficult and somewhat painful to do.

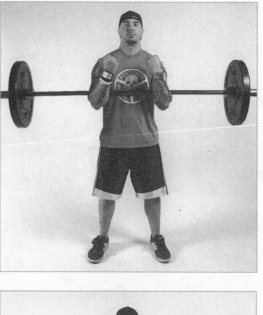

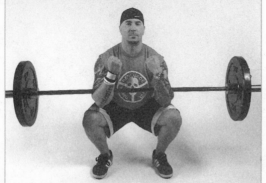

Single Leg Squat

Unilateral leg work is great for all combat athletes, as mixed martial arts involves transferring power from one limb to the other. Single-limb training also helps correct imbalances and prevent injuries. Stand on a box or bench with one leg hanging off the side. Squat down as low as you can on your working leg, keeping your nonworking leg hanging down or, if possible, extended in front of you in the "pistol" position.

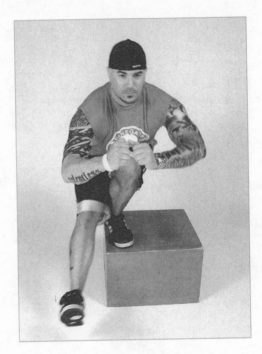

Split Squat

Split your legs so that one is a few feet in front of the other (like you've just taken a step). Keeping your torso upright, bend both knees and lower your body, squatting down and slightly forward with the front leg. Your hamstring on your front leg should touch your calf on the same leg. Now straighten both knees to raise yourself back to the starting position. This also can be done while holding dumbbells or with your back foot elevated on a bench to increase the challenge to your balance.

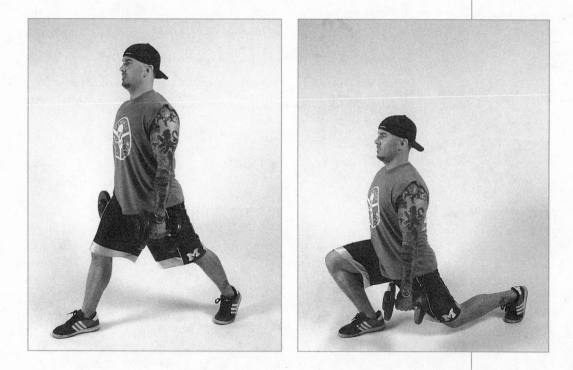

Lunge

Step forward as far as you comfortably can while maintaining perfectly upright posture. Push explosively off of your front leg to return to the start position, and then switch legs. Continue to alternate legs until you finish all of the prescribed reps. This is a great exercise because it simulates the type of move you make when you shoot in on an opponent.

Dead Lift

The dead lift is probably the single greatest size- and strength-building exercise there is. Dead lifts work your traps, upper back, lats, lower back, biceps, forearms, glutes, hamstrings, and quads. If you could only choose one exercise, this would be the one. No other exercise will be as effective in giving you the strength and power needed for combat.

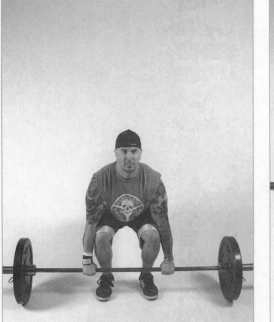
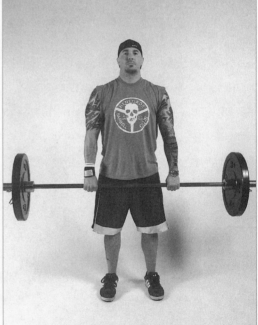

A proper dead lift begins with the correct bar placement, grip width, and stance width. Load the barbell and set it on the floor. Stand with the bar about an inch away from your shins, your stance slightly narrower than shoulder width.

Squat down and grab the bar with an overhand shoulder-width grip. Keep your head straight and your back tightly arched. Start the lift by pulling up and back toward you, making sure to get a strong leg drive. Once the bar is past your knees, push your hips forward. Return to the starting position by sitting back and then lowering the bar, trying not to squat down until the bar clears your knees. Let the plates touch the ground and repeat.

Do not allow your hips to rise before your shoulders and upper body. Doing this turns the exercise into more of a stiff-legged dead lift, is very stressful on your back, and puts you in a weaker position. Let your shoulders and hips come up at the same time and pace.

Although the dead lift is the best exercise there is, it also has its draw-backs. Dead lifting is extremely stressful on the body and the central nervous system. As a beginner, you might be able to dead lift three times a week, but as you get more advanced and pull more weight, you should decrease the frequency. Intermediates can get away with dead lifting once a week, while more-advanced lifters would be better served to only dead lift once every 10 to 21 days.

Rack Dead Lift

This is a standard dead lift performed off pins in a power rack. The pins can be set anywhere from an inch off the ground all the way up to lower thigh height. The higher you set the pins, the more weight you will be able to lift. These will do wonders for your upper, middle, and lower back development. The highest starting position you should use for a rack dead lift is about 3 to 4 inches above the knee. Using a higher starting position than this is a major mistake, because it allows you to use too much weight and puts your back at risk of injury.

Romanian Dead Lift

Load a barbell and set it on the floor. Stand over it with your feet at shoulder width, and grab the bar with an overhand grip. Keeping an extremely tight arch in your lower back, and your knees slightly bent,

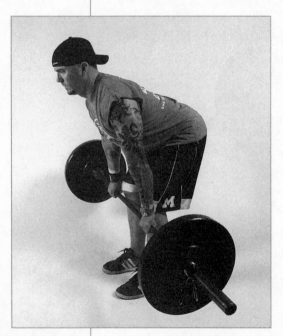

lift the bar while sticking your glutes straight back and out as far as you can. Make sure to keep your chest out and your shoulder blades squeezed together. Descend until your upper body is parallel with the floor, and then return to the starting position by explosively pushing your hips forward and squeezing your glutes.

Good Morning

Load a barbell and set it on your traps (lower than if you were squatting). Your grip will be wider than what you use for a squat as well. The Good Morning is basically a Romanian dead lift with the bar on your back, and thus the execution is exactly the same. Initiate the movement by breaking at the hips and pushing your glutes out as far as you can. Making sure to keep your back arched and your head in line with your spine, bend your torso until you are slightly above parallel to the floor. If you are doing Good Mornings for the sole purpose of improving your squat, then you needn't go lower than 45 degrees, because that is as bent forward as you will ever find yourself in a squat. Make sure to grip the bar tightly to avoid having it roll forward when you go down. To return to the start position, powerfully drive your hips forward and stand upright.

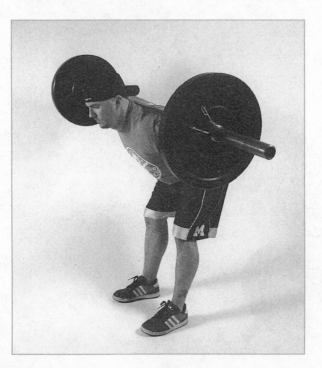

45-Degree Back Extension

Position yourself on the apparatus so that your hips are completely off the end of the pad. Lower your upper body by breaking at the hips, keeping your back arched. You can increase the difficulty by holding a weight on your chest or, when that gets too easy, putting a bar on your back.

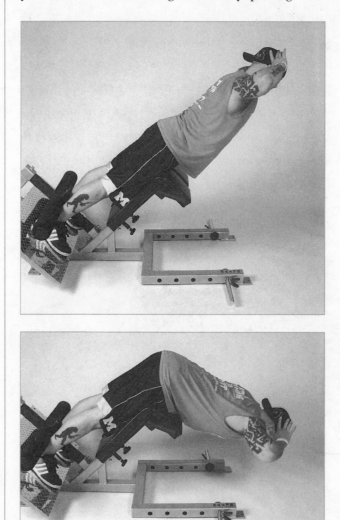

Glute Ham Raise

This is one of the greatest pure hamstring movements you can do. You need a dedicated bench for this exercise (the best ones on the market are available at EliteFTS.com). Hook your legs between the ankle pads and straighten your body so that you are parallel with the floor. Begin by driving your toes into the plate and push your knees into the pad while pulling as hard as you can with your hamstrings. To make this easier, you can start at a position below parallel to gain some momentum when you come up. You can also allow your knees to drop a little bit as you come up. To increase the difficulty, hold a weight on your chest or behind your head.

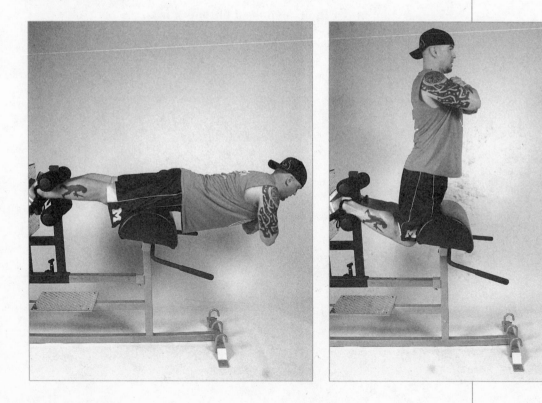

Dumbbell Swing

Hold a dumbbell with one hand and bend down by pushing your hips back as far as you can. At the start position you should be in a half-squat with the dumbbell between your legs. Begin the movement by popping your hips forward and standing up straight. The dumbbell should swing forward and ascend to eye level. At the top, your hips should be completely straightened and you should be on your toes. Be sure to control the weight on the way down and keep your shoulders firmly locked in the sockets. Allow the weight to swing all the way through your legs before repeating the next rep. The trick here is to use the momentum from your explosive hip drive to move the weight—be careful not to just turn the movement into a Romanian dead lift plus a front raise.

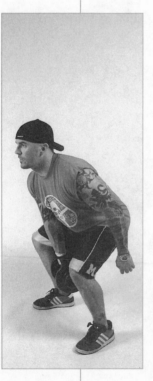
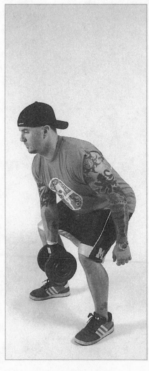
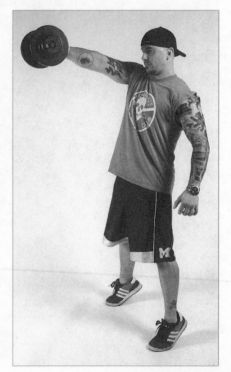

Neck Extension with Harness and Plate

Having a strong neck is critically important to all mixed martial artists. It literally could be the difference between serious injury and victory. Much description is not necessary for this exercise. Simply attach a plate to the harness, put the harness over your head, sit down with your forearms resting on your quads, and move your head up and down while keeping your back arched. Make sure not to use extreme ranges of motion, i.e., don't go down too low and come up too high by jamming your head all the way back into your traps.

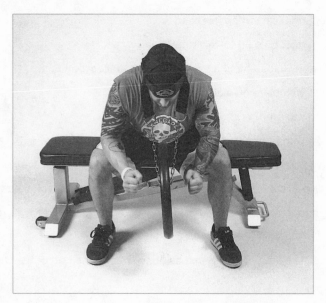

- **How often should a combat athlete be training his neck, and what are some good exercises?**

- Neck work is of the utmost importance for the combat athlete, and the neck should be trained at least twice a week. Some great neck exercises include:

  - Neck Extension with harness and plate
  - Neck Extension with harness and band
  - Neck Extension with harness and cable
  - Neck Flexion with plate on forehead
  - Neck Flexion with partner's hand on forehead
  - Neck Flexion with partner holding towel on forehead
  - Isometric Neck Flexion Holds—Hold anywhere from 8 to 30 seconds
  - Lateral Neck Flexion with plate on side of head
  - Lateral Neck Flexion with partner's hand on forehead
  - Lateral Neck Flexion with partner holding towel on forehead
  - Isometric Lateral Neck Flexion—Hold anywhere from 8 to 30 seconds
  - Neck Support on Swiss Ball—Place a Swiss ball against a wall and lean your forehead into the ball, supporting all your weight with your neck, and hold for 30 to 60 seconds
  - Neck Support on Glute Ham Bench—Same as above but on the pad of the Glute Ham Bench
  - Neck Bridge on Swiss Ball—Lie down on a Swiss ball and roll out so that only the back of your head is on the ball, supporting your body weight with your neck, making sure to keep your hips up, parallel with the ground

The sets, reps, and frequency prescribed for neck work are dependent on how often you train your neck. Most combat athletes would be best served to start by training the neck with 2 to 3 sets twice a week. From there you can increase the frequency to 3 to 4 times a week, and eventually you may want to try doing 1 to 2 sets every day. Frequently switch up the exercises and vary the way you do them. And be sure to keep the reps fairly high on most neck work. Unless, of course, you are doing isometric holds. Below is an example of how to train the neck 6 days a week while varying the exercises and rep ranges.

Monday: Neck Harness: 1–2 x 15

Tuesday: Lateral Flexion with partner: 1–2 x 20

Wednesday: Neck Flexion with plate:1–2 x 25

Thursday: Neck Bridge on Swiss Ball: 1–2 x 30 seconds

Friday: Isometric Lateral Neck Flexion: 1–2 x 8 (hold each rep for 6 seconds)

Saturday: Neck Support on Swiss Ball: 1–2 x 60 seconds

Manual Resistance Neck Flexion

You'll need a partner and a towel for the next three exercises. While lying faceup on a standard bench, have a partner place a towel over your forehead and provide resistance as you move your head up and down.

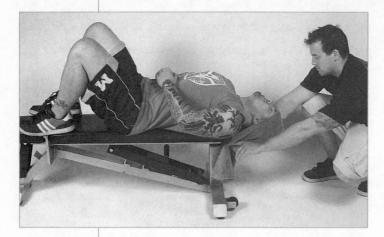

Manual Resistance Neck Extension

While lying facedown on a standard bench, have your partner place the towel over the back of your head and provide resistance as you move your head up and down.

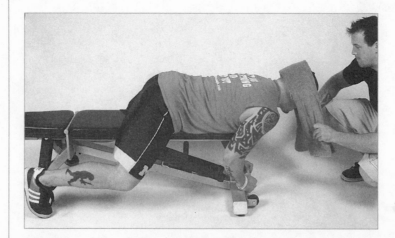

Manual Resistance Lateral Neck Flexion

Lie on your side with your head hanging off the end of a bench and have your partner drape the towel over your head, providing resistance as you move your head up and down.

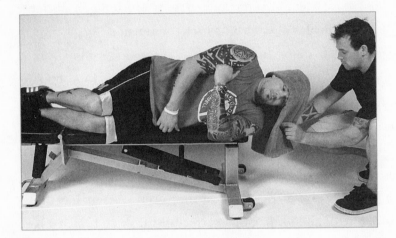

Rear Neck Support on Swiss Ball

Lay the back of your head on a Swiss ball while keeping your body straight and parallel with the ground. Roll out far enough so that just your head is on the ball and most of your body weight is being supported by your neck. Hold this position as long as you can. To increase the difficulty, hold a weight on your chest.

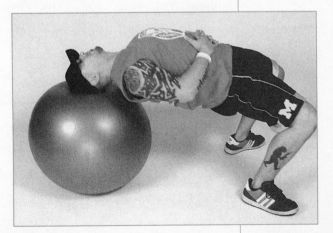

Training for Speed

When we talk about training for speed we mean using the dynamic effort method. This method involves lifting light to moderate loads with a focus on speed and acceleration. The goal of this method is to stimulate the central nervous system to improve the rate at which it recruits muscle fibers and coordinates a powerful muscle contraction.

Included here are jumps, throws, catches, absorption drills, Olympic lifts, and high-speed lifting with a relatively light weight (45 to 60 percent of 1RM). For throws, I usually use medicine balls or in some cases barbells or kettlebells. The weights used on these types of exercises should also be relatively light (10 to 25 percent of your 1RM). Your focus should be on speed and technique, not on heavy weight.

Often a throwing exercise is also a catching exercise. You may throw a medicine ball back and forth with a partner or throw and catch a barbell yourself, such as in the ballistic bench press. These catches are called absorption drills, and are of great importance to combat athletes because you must be able to successfully absorb your opponent's force when he makes a move on you. When you're in the middle of a fight, you often have to absorb force rapidly before quickly turning the tide and generating force in the opposite direction. Absorption drills are great training for what you'll face in the cage.

Olympic lifting, the snatches and clean and jerks you see in the Olympics, is becoming very popular among mixed martial artists. All the Olympic lifts are total-body exercises and require you to produce force at a rapid rate. The majority of Olympic lifts also have some kind of pulling component, which is beneficial, since most upper body movement in mat sports is based on pulling.

I'm going to show you how to lift relatively light weights explosively in order to improve your rate of force production—your explosive speed. The weights used for these exercises usually will be between 45 and 60 percent of your 1 rep max for the given lift. Exercises such as squats and overhead presses can be used with this method to achieve outstanding results.

These are what I consider the best speed-training exercises:

Hang Snatch

Grab a bar with an overhand grip, placing your index fingers on the outer rings. Stand up and bend over so that the bar is just above your knees, making sure your back is arched, chest is up, butt is out, and elbows are straight. Initiate the movement by popping your hips forward and shrugging as high as you can. As the bar moves its way up your thighs and approaches hip height, extend your knees and get up on the balls of your feet while pulling the bar straight up as high as you can.

When the bar is at eye level, flip it up and over your head. As you are flipping the bar up to lockout in the overhead position, dip under it slightly, so that you catch the bar's momentum and finish in a quarter-squat position.

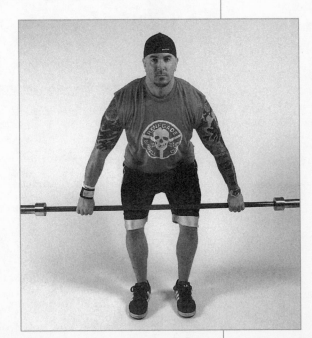

Hang Clean

Load the bar and grab it with a shoulder-width overhand grip. Stand up and, keeping your lower back in its natural arch, bend at the hips so that the bar touches the front of your thighs, just above your knees. Squeeze your shoulder blades together, stick your chest out, and keep your head up. Explosively pop your hips forward and shrug your shoulders, generating momentum so that the bar begins to rise straight up in front of you. As the bar passes your abdomen, pull up as high as you can, come up on the balls of your feet, and flip your wrists over so that you catch the bar at shoulder level. You should finish with your upper arms parallel to the floor.

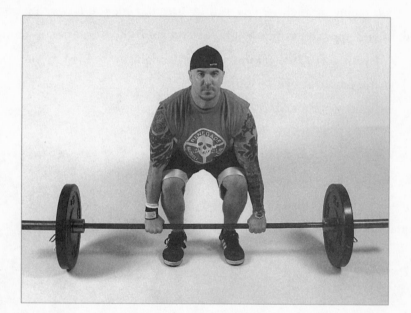

Hang Clean and Jerk

Begin this exercise by performing the Hang Clean as described on page 132. From the catch position, lower your body into a quarter-squat, and then immediately drive with your legs to explosively come back up and press the weight straight overhead. As you're coming up, split your legs so that one goes in front and the other behind you as in a lunge. This must be done as quickly as possible, so use light weights, and concentrate on speed.

Box Jump

You will need a box for this, one that you can safely jump up and land on. Set it about 6 to 12 inches in front of you, and with a quick, powerful dip, jump straight up onto the box. Step down and repeat.

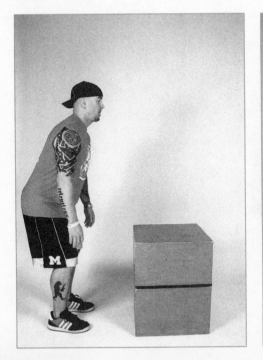
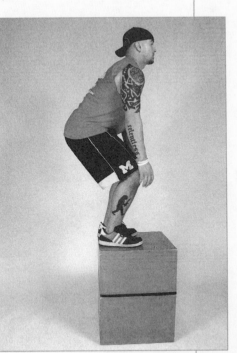

Hurdle Jump

This is performed just like a box jump, except instead of landing on the box you simply jump over it like a hurdle.

Depth Jump

This is an advanced speed and plyometric exercise. You will need two boxes for this exercise, placed roughly three feet apart. To perform the exercise, stand on one box, then step off and land on both feet with minimal knee flexion. As quickly as you can (pretend the ground is on fire), jump onto the other box or jump it as a hurdle. To increase the difficulty of this exercise, increase the height of the boxes but never so much that your ground contact time increases. Jumps usually should be kept to 6 reps or fewer per set.

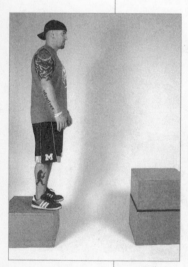 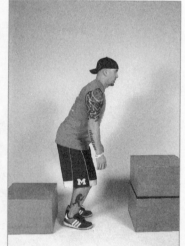 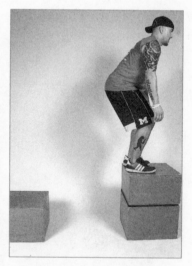

Jump Squat

Start with a weight that is 15 percent of your 1 rep max on a regular squat. Descend halfway down and, without pausing, explode up and jump as high as you can. Catch yourself and quickly reset before the next rep.

Box Squat

As described on page 113.

Medicine Ball Overhead Throw

It's a good idea to do the medicine ball exercises outside or somewhere with enough space for hurling the ball. Hold the ball over your head like you would in a sideline throw in soccer. Take a step forward and throw the ball as far as you can.

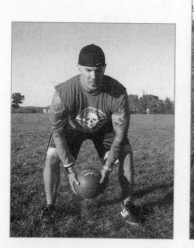
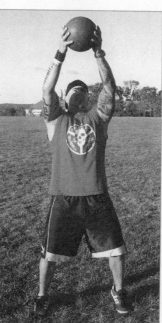
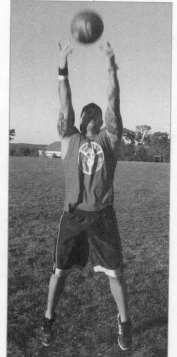

Medicine Ball Chest Pass

Hold a medicine ball with both hands at chest height and step forward while throwing the ball as hard and as fast as possible. You can throw the ball to a partner (who then throws it back to you) or into a wall and catch it.

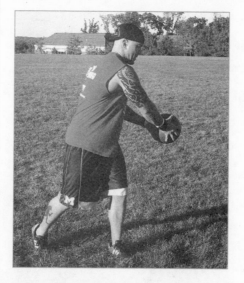

Medicine Ball Rotational Side Throw

You'll need a partner for this exercise. Stand sideways about 5 feet away from your partner. As he throws the ball to you, catch the ball with both hands extended in front of you. Rotate to the side and then use your obliques to explosively throw the ball back as hard as you can.

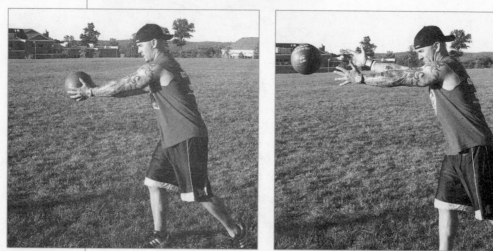

One-Arm Overhead Kettlebell Throw

Perform this like a dumbbell swing, but bring the kettlebell all the way up until your arm is directly over your head. Then release the weight, throwing it as far as possible. Be sure to explode and actually jump off the ground when you release the weight.

Plyo Push-up

This is a great exercise for developing explosive strength and speed in the shoulders, chest, and triceps. A plyo push-up is simply a push-up in which you propel your hands off the floor on each and every rep.

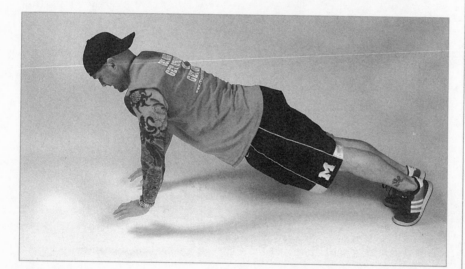

Depth Push-up

You'll need two low boxes for this exercise. Get into a push-up position with your hands on two low boxes. Let your hands quickly drop off the boxes, and as soon as you touch the ground, bend your elbows and explosively push yourself back up onto the boxes. Repeat for the prescribed reps.

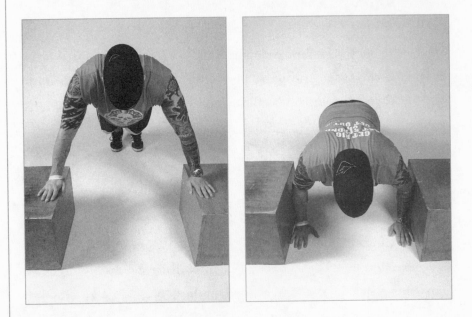

Sandbag Rotational Side Throw

Grab a sandbag and stand straight up with it at arm's length. Rotate to one side to generate momentum and then explosively rotate in the opposite direction with a powerful contraction of the obliques. As you reach full extension, release the bag while attempting to throw it as far as possible.

Overhead Keg Throw

See description in the strongman section, page 70.

Putting It All Together

All three of the methods discussed above—the max effort, repeated effort, and dynamic effort—must be integrated into a comprehensive program that prevents plateaus and allows you to make ongoing progress. Most coaches try to accomplish this in one of two ways. The first way is known as Western periodization, or linear periodization, and it remains one of the most widely used systems in the country. In fact, if you worked with a strength coach during your high school or college athletic career, you likely trained according to some kind of linear model. Western periodization takes the three methods of strength training explained in this chapter and breaks them down into separate training phases. So, for example, a typical Western scheme might have you perform a four- to six-week strength and hypertrophy (muscle-building) block where you focus predominantly on the repeated-effort method and try to maximize your muscular size. After that, you might move into a pure strength block for the next four to six weeks, focusing on heavy weights and using the max-effort method. Upon completion of that phase, you would then move into a speed phase where you used the dynamic-effort method almost exclusively for improving speed and power.

The problem with this type of system is that when you go longer than two weeks without training a specific skill, you begin to lose the progress you made! That means that when you finish your hypertrophy (muscle-building) phase and enter your strength phase, your muscular size may begin to diminish in only two weeks. When another two to four more weeks pass, you will lose even more size. Then you will begin your speed phase, stronger but smaller. Within a few weeks you will start to lose the strength you gained during your max-effort phase and your muscular size will still be plummeting. Now, when you finally finish your speed phase, you may be faster, but you are also smaller and weaker—not a good scenario.

There's got to be a better way, you say. Luckily for all of us, there is. Enter the conjugate method of periodization. The conjugate method involves training all strength qualities simultaneously throughout the yearly training plan. This means that all three methods are constantly used, and that all strength qualities are constantly improving. Though it's not foolproof, it is an excellent way for all athletes to train.

So how exactly do we go about doing it? I have experimented with these parameters with hundreds of athletes over the years. I have tried every way possible of combining these methods to bring about optimal results. For the purpose of training combat athletes, I have found one particular way of combining these methods that works better than all the others, which I will lay out for you here.

Day 1: Maximal-Effort Day
Day 2: Dynamic-Effort Day
Day 3: Repeated-Effort/Strongman Training Day

On the following pages, you will find a sample workout along with exercise descriptions.

On most exercises, except for dynamic or explosive lifts, you should control the eccentric or lowering portion of the exercise and perform the concentric or lifting portion of the exercise as explosively as possible. On dynamic-effort exercises or Olympic lifts there is no controlled eccentric—the entire movement should be explosive.

I use full-body workouts for several reasons. The days of training one body part per day are dead. The notion that a body part should only be trained once a week started in bodybuilding circles some time in the seventies. This theory was never intended to find its way into the training programs of athletes. Somehow it did, but the time to end it is right now. Athletes train for performance, not for looks, and performance gains are based on high frequency, not high volume. In Eastern European countries such as Russia and Bulgaria, Olympic lifters perform up to eighteen low-volume workouts a week with the goal of improving the snatch and the clean and jerk. Historically, these lifters have dominated the Olympics, a fact that speaks volumes about the importance of high frequency. Improving strength involves improving the efficacy of the nervous system. To do this, you need to expose your body to the stimulus on a frequent basis.

To simplify this point, I ask you this question: If you wanted to improve your techniques on the mat, would you practice them only once a week? Of course you wouldn't. So how then can you expect to improve your lifts by doing the same? For performance gains, you must train each movement pattern at least twice a week, with three times usually being optimal. Because combat sports are so demanding and involve long hours of practice, it usually is better to stick with three workouts a week. Don't risk overtraining by pushing it to five times a week.

PHASE 1

DAY 1

Exercise	Sets	Reps	Rest (seconds)
(1a) Dumbbell Split Squat	2	10–12	90
(1b) One-Arm Dumbbell Row	2	10–12	90
(2a) 45-Degree Back Extension	2	15–20	90
(2b) Blast Strap Push-up	2	Amap*	90
(3a) Face Pull	2	12–15	90
(3b) Side Plank	2	Alap*	90
(4) Neck Harness Extension	2	20–25	90

DAY 2

Exercise	Sets	Reps	Rest
(1a) Chin-up	3	6–8	90
(1b) Dumbbell Step-up	3	6–8	90
(2) One-Arm Standing Cable Press	3	6–8	90
(3a) Plank	3	Alap*	90
(3b) Dumbbell Shrug	2	8–10	90
(4) Manual Resistance Neck Flexion	2	15–20	90

DAY 3

Exercise	Sets	Reps	Rest
(1) Forward Sled Drag	2	100 feet	180
(2) Backward Sled Drag	2	100 feet	180
(3) Sandbag Hang Clean	2	8–10	180
(4) Standing Sandbag Press	2	8–10	180
(5) Farmers Walk	2	200 feet	180

*Amap=as many as possible
*Alap=as long as possible

PHASE 2

DAY 1

Exercise	Sets	Reps	Rest
(1) Box Squat	2	6	180
(2a) Parallel Chin-up	2	6	90
(2b) One-Arm Flat Dumbbell Press	2	6	90
(3) Modified Turkish Get-up	2	6	90
(4) Manual Resistance Lateral Neck Flexion	2	12	90

DAY 2

Exercise	Sets	Reps	Rest
(1) Box Jump	3	5	120
(2) Jump Squat	3	10	120
(3) One-Arm Dumbbell or Kettlebell Snatch	3	6	120
(4) Medicine Ball Chest Pass	4	6	90
(5) Rear Neck Support on Swiss Ball	2	30 seconds	90

DAY 3

Exercise	Sets	Reps	Rest
(1) Prowler/Car Push	2	50 feet	180
(2) Rope Row	2	50 feet	180
(3) Standing Keg Press	2	8–10	180
(4) Sandbag Zercher Carry	2	300 feet	180
(5) Dumbbell Hand Walk	2	50–100 feet	180

PHASE 3

DAY 1

Exercise	Sets	Reps	Rest
(1) Squat/Dead Lift	3	4–5	180
(2a) Incline Dumbbell Press	3	4–5	90
(2b) Pull-up	3	4–5	90
(3a) Hanging Knee Raise	3	6–10	60
(3b) Manual Resistance Neck Flexion	2	10–12	60

DAY 2

Exercise	Sets	Reps	Rest
(1) Depth Jump	4	3	120
(2) Hang Snatch	4	3	90
(3) Push Press	4	3	120
(4) Rotational Side Medicine Ball Throw	3	5	120
(5a) Neck Harness Extension	2	12–15	60
(5b) Incline Y Raise	2	8–10	60

DAY 3

Exercise	Sets	Reps	Rest
(1) Keg Clean and Press	2	6–8	150
(2) Tire Flip	2	6–8	180
(3) Sandbag Zercher Walking Lunge	2	6–8	180
(4) Overhead Sledgehammer Swing	2	8–10	120
(5) Sandbag Rotational Side Throw	2	6–8	180

PHASE 4

DAY 1

Exercise	Sets	Reps	Rest
(1) Squat/Dead Lift	3	2–3	180
(2a) Towel Chin-up	3	2–3	90
(2b) Flat Dumbbell Press	3	2–3	90
(3a) Barbell Russian Twist	3	4–5	75
(3b) Neck Harness Extension	2	8–10	75

DAY 2

Exercise	Sets	Reps	Rest
(1) Hurdle Jump	5	3	90
(2) Hang Clean	5	2	120
(3) Depth Push-up	5	3	90
(4) Medicine Ball Overhead Soccer Throw	5	3	90
(5) Manual Resistance Lateral Neck Flexion	2	8–10	90

DAY 3

Exercise	Sets	Reps	Rest
(1) Overhead Keg Throw	2	4	150
(2) Prowler/Sled Backward Drag	2	100 feet	180
(3) Tire Flip	2	5	180
(4) Rope Row	2	50 feet	180
(5) Sandbag Shouldering	2	5–7 per side	120 between sides

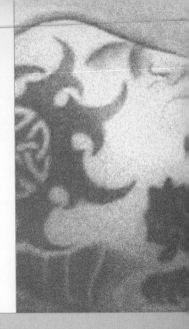

6 COMBAT NUTRITION: FOOD TO FIGHT

THE OTHER DAY, AS I WAS CHANNEL SURFING, I CAME ACROSS AN
episode of a mixed martial arts reality show. I was shocked to see that in
order to "make weight," these athletes were using last-minute, old-
school dehydration methods that not only can hinder performance, but
can be dangerous as well. These athletes were running while wearing rubber suiting, chewing gum, and spitting out all of their saliva, sitting in a
sauna without drinking any fluid, vomiting, and perhaps the most haz-
ardous of all, using diuretics. In addition to possibly killing you, all these
techniques will sap your strength and weaken your performance. Over the
past few decades, these unhealthy training techniques have cost some incredibly talented young collegiate wrestlers their lives. Rather than have
you risk going down that road, I'm going to show you how to control your
weight with good nutrition that will optimize your performance while
keeping you healthy. I have found that, by and large, grappling and
mixed martial arts are still in the dark ages of nutrition. For instance, the

antiquated and dangerous methods of dehydration mentioned above have been passed down from coach to athlete in a seemingly never-ending cycle. From years of working with athletes, I've never ceased to be shocked that so many wrestlers and grapplers still rely on these unhealthy, last-minute methods of losing weight. And, because they are accustomed to this "cramming" method of losing weight, they tend not to be disciplined with their diet year-round. In other words, they are occasionally dropping weight in an unhealthy fashion, and the rest of the time they are eating junk food. So they are not only exposing themselves to the dangers of excessive last-minute dehydration, they are also missing the performance and recovery benefits of a sound, healthy, year-round nutrition program. Well, it's time to break that cycle with a serious paradigm shift.

In this chapter, I teach you how to maintain a weight closer to your fighting weight by using proper nutritional strategies. This doesn't mean that you will simply eat less year-round to keep your weight down. On the contrary, because of the nature of the training necessary to succeed in this sport, your calorie requirements are, in fact, relatively high. By following my plan, your energy levels will soar, your recovery times will be shorter, your body fat percentage will drop, and your performance will improve. You will also avoid last-minute panicking, excessive dehydration, and unnecessary performance interference. To accomplish all of these goals while simultaneously taking your performance to the next level, we must consider food quality, activity levels, nutrient timing, food combining, blood-sugar levels, calorie requirements, your current body fat percentage, training intensity, and more. To discuss all of these in detail is beyond the scope of this book. But you don't need a nutrition textbook to get the best useable dietary advice. I've distilled the essence here, which you'll find easy to follow and almost foolproof.

Guideline #1: Calorie Requirements

First and foremost, you must figure out how many calories you should be consuming daily. For this we will use a very simple formula: Simply multiply your body weight by 18. This will give you a good baseline daily caloric intake. Other factors also determine calorie requirements, including metabolism, lifestyle, and body-weight goals. Full-time fighters who train up to six hours a day during training camp prior to a big fight will have specific calorie requirements. Because I'm not working with you directly, you must make adjustments on your own. Just use this formula to start with and, if necessary, adjust your calories up or down 300 calories at a time. If you are gaining body fat, subtract 300 calories a day; if you are feeling lethargic, lacking energy during your workouts, or losing muscle mass, then increase your calories by 300 a day. Give this new adjustment a week's trial run and assess your progress. If you are still not satisfied with your progress, continue to increase or decrease your calories by 300 a day until you reach the optimal caloric intake for you.

Guideline #2: Increase Your Meal Frequency

Eating frequently is one of the best ways to simultaneously build muscle and lose fat. This is because frequent feedings keep a steady supply of muscle-building nutrients in your bloodstream and also elevate your metabolism, forcing you to burn more fat throughout the day. You should consume a meal (solid or liquid) every 2½ to 3 hours. By doing this, you will eat between 5 and 7 meals daily. In order to figure out the calories you should eat per meal, just take your total number of calories and divide that by the total number of meals you decide to eat daily.

- **Why is it so important for mixed martial artists to possess such low levels of body fat?**

- Because excess fat does two things: It slows you down and it hurts your endurance. There is absolutely no need to be carrying excess body fat in combat sports. First, that excess baggage will slow you down every time you throw a strike. And second, lugging around excess body fat is exhausting and draining. Body fat is nonfunctional tissue with little purpose.

  Your goal should be to be as lean as your opponent but with more muscle mass. For example, if your opponent weighs 205 at 16% body fat, he has 172.2 pounds of lean body mass. If you also weigh 205 but are 6% body fat, you have 192.7 pounds of lean body mass. That means you are actually more than 20 pounds bigger than your opponent in the same weight class!

Let's say our 200-pounder decides to eat six meals daily.

$$3960/6 = 660 \text{ calories per meal}$$

If you are not already eating your meals with this type of frequency, then this simple change alone will work wonders for you. In combat sports, you want to be as strong as possible for your body weight. One very desirable side effect of increasing your meal frequency is that it will boost your metabolic rate, thus inducing that much-sought-after fat loss. It is important to remember that fat is noncontractile tissue. Unlike muscle, it doesn't do anything to contribute to your performance in a positive way . . . so let the fat go!

An additional benefit of eating frequent meals is increased stability in your energy levels, thus allowing you to train more intensely, more consistently, and more frequently.

The next question we need to answer is: Where should these calories come from? Any good muscle-building diet begins with protein.

Guideline #3: Build Your Meals Around a Base of Protein

You'll need approximately 1 gram of protein per pound of body weight daily. Only count protein from complete sources, such as lean meats, fish, and cottage cheese. Do not include the small amount of protein found in some of your carb sources. (See the 10 Percent Rule, page 155 for more on this.)

You need a steady flow of amino acids in your bloodstream throughout the day. Amino acids are simply the building blocks of protein. When your protein intake is inadequate for your energy needs, your body pulls amino acids from your muscles as needed, resulting in catabolism (muscle breakdown). Obviously, you're training to build strength and mass, not to lose it, so you have to feed your muscles to both get stronger and avoid breakdown. During a strenuous mixed martial arts training session, your tissues will break down. You need protein for the formation of new tissues, so be sure to include a quality protein source at every meal.

Below are the best sources of protein:

Whole eggs
Egg whites
Fat-free or low-fat cheese
Fat-free or low-fat cottage cheese

Chicken

Turkey

Canned tuna

Canned chicken

Lean ground beef

Steak

Buffalo meat

Ostrich meat

Venison

Lamb

Veal

Salmon

Tuna

Swordfish

Shrimp

Lobster

Crabmeat

Protein powder (see Chapter 7, "Supplements," for a discussion of the
best and worst protein powders)

Guideline #4: Include a Vegetable Source at Every Meal Except Breakfast and Post-Workout

Even though most athletes pay attention to their total protein and caloric
intake, often their vegetable intake is an afterthought at best. In fact,
over the years I've noticed that many athletes eat no vegetables at all. Vegetables are great for your overall health. They provide important vitamins
and minerals, fiber, enzymes, and a small amount of clean carbohy-

drates. Adding vegetables to a meal also will slow the entry rate of carbohydrates into the bloodstream. This in turn will modify insulin output to favor muscle maintenance and building while simultaneously encouraging fat burning. The only times I exclude vegetables from a meal are at breakfast and post-workout. This is because vegetables contain fiber, which slows down the absorption of nutrients. During breakfast and the post-workout period you want nutrients to be absorbed rapidly. These are the two times when your glycogen levels are low and need quick replenishment. While there are many vegetables to choose from, look for those that are dark in color, as they contain the most nutrients. Examples include broccoli, kale, asparagus, green beans, and spinach.

Guideline #5: Replenish Yourself with Post-Workout Nutrition

After a brutal MMA workout, your muscle's energy stores will be severely depleted. While tissue damage sounds harsh, in fact it's a necessary step toward a stronger body. Your body will adapt and grow, but only if you first recover from your workouts. The greatest recovery tool is a post-workout shake, consumed right after training.

A well-prepared shake provides the raw materials that your muscles need for replenishment. Your recovery shake should include both protein and fast-acting carbs. So you'll want a protein-carb combo that contains hydrolyzed whey protein and maltodextrin or waxy maize (read the label). To calculate how many carbs to consume in this shake, simply take your body weight in pounds and multiply it by 0.5. After many years of experimentation I have found this to be the optimal ratio.

For your post-workout shake, carbohydrates that are easy to digest are superior to slower-acting natural carbs. These simple carbs will rapidly replenish muscle-glycogen stores. The reason I suggest malto-dextrin powder, a derivative of corn, is that it's cheap and readily available on Internet supplement sites and health food stores. As for your protein, just take your body weight and multiply it by 0.25. I like to use whey protein. Whey is rapidly digested and absorbed by the body, and it contains all the essential amino acids. Don't buy into the hype that you need some scientifically engineered formula to best replenish your body. I've tried them all, and this combination works just as well, for a fraction of the cost. Do not include any fat in your post-workout shake. This will decrease its effectiveness by slowing down the absorption of the carbs and protein during this period. Although fats are detrimental immediately post-workout, consuming the right types of fats is extremely important. This brings us to our next guideline.

Guideline #6: Consume an Adequate Amount of Fatty Acids, Except During Your Post-Workout Meal

Fats have been demonized, yet who among us doesn't love them? For many of us, fat is a hidden vice, a shameful indulgence on par with hard drugs or Everclear. But not all fats are harmful, and many are essential for our health and well-being. The saturated fats found in red meats or full-fat cheese are wildly different from the fats found in salmon or walnuts. Some fats are even called essential because the body needs them to survive. In particular, omega-3 fatty acids are highly effective in decreasing body fat by improving insulin sensitivity. Furthermore, fats play an extremely important role in energy metabolism and all bodily functions. Omega-3s also provide powerful anti-inflammatory benefits, another plus for combat fighters.

More and more nutritionists and doctors are recommending omega-3s, but usually in less-than-optimal doses. Athletes, and especially combat fighters, need at least 3 grams per 100 pounds of body weight daily. You can use fish oil capsules or flaxseed oil (1 tablespoon flaxseed oil per 100 pounds of body weight). I usually have my athletes alternate between the two.

We recently have learned of the dangers of trans fats, which are the partially hydrogenated fats and oils found in everything from fast food french fries to microwave popcorn to most store-bought cookies. In fact, the whole processed-food industry was built on trans fats. These fats, not found in nature, extend the shelf life of foods (unlike butter or natural oils, which spoil quickly). So these fats were designed to benefit the food industry, not you. Like saturated fats, they clog your arteries, increase inflammation, and make you much more susceptible to diabetes and heart disease. Always read the labels on the food you eat. Trans fats are usually listed as partially hydrogenated vegetable oil or shortening.

To determine your daily fat intake, take your total daily calories and multiply by 0.25. Then divide the resulting number by 9 (fat has 9 calories per gram). This will tell you how many grams of fat you should consume daily. Good fat sources include almonds, walnuts, avocados, pistachios, and olive oil.

Guideline #7: Carbohydrate Intake and the 10 Percent Rule

When people say simple carbs, they're usually talking about the kind that burn up quickly in your body, giving you a short burst of energy followed by a long period of feeling like crap. You're already familiar with most of these—pasta, white rice, and almost any other sugary, doughy, or white food you can think of. These foods enter the bloodstream quickly and elicit an aggressive insulin response, and that encourages the body to store a greater percentage of that blood sugar as body fat. But simple carbs also include fruits and many vegetables.

Complex carbs, on the other hand, are the ones that burn slowly, giving you lasting energy for a prolonged period without putting you to sleep afterward. These carbs are more likely to be stored as muscle glycogen, the main source of fuel for training and fighting. They include oatmeal, potatoes, yams, and brown rice, to name a few. Including a fibrous vegetable in each meal (see Guideline #4) also helps mitigate insulin's effects on your body, transferring carbohydrate to muscle glycogen rather than to fat.

As discussed earlier, simple fast-burning carbs aren't all bad, and can even be highly beneficial (as in the morning and immediately post-workout). Most of your carb intake should be vegetables, fruits, and the complex kind such as yams and oatmeal. Skip the carbs found in refined foods, such as doughnuts or cookies.

Now we'll determine how many calories you need to eat, and how to divvy them up over the course of the day.

Carbohydrates should make up 50 percent of your total daily calories. To determine how many grams of carbs you should eat each day, simply multiply your total daily calorie intake by .5 and then divide this number by 4.

With your daily carb tally determined, here's how those carbs should be portioned throughout the day:

On training days, take your total daily grams of carbs and divide by 6. Call this amount "1 serving" of carbs. Your post-workout meal should contain 1.5 of these "servings." Every other meal will be 1 serving, except for your last meal of the day, which will contain .5 serving. That way, you finish off your day with a slightly diminished portion of carbohydrates.

On nontraining days, simply have 1 serving at each meal.

Below is a list of the best carbohydrate sources:

Oatmeal

Whole wheat bread

White potatoes

Quinoa

Sweet potatoes

Brown rice

Hot oat bran cereal

Apples

Oranges

Pears

Plums

Peaches

Melons

Blueberries

Blackberries

Strawberries

Raspberries

Bell peppers

String beans

Spinach

Broccoli

Cauliflower

Carrots

Tomatoes

Beans

Guideline #8: Don't Mix Large Amounts of Carbohydrates and Fats in the Same Meal

It's the American way: carbs and fat, fat and carbs. All of our "favorite" foods contain this lethal combination: pizza, ice cream, cheeseburgers, and donuts. The common thread is that all are fat/carb delivery systems. Fast, easy, cheap, and terrible for you. Stick with meals consisting of either protein and fat or protein and carbs, not fat and carbs. Consume the bulk of your carbohydrates in the early morning or after a training session. If you are a professional MMA athlete and are pretty much training all day, you can get away with breaking this rule. For your energy demands, it would be impossible to follow this rule and eat as much as you need to perform at your highest capacity. Just don't go overboard and mix saturated fats with sugar; that is the worst combo in existence.

Guideline #9: Base Your Diet Around Natural, Organic, Whole-Food Sources

The majority of your calories should come from organic meats, eggs, nuts, legumes, fruits, and vegetables. To simplify this point, I always tell my clients that if a caveman couldn't eat it, then you shouldn't eat it. Avoid most packaged or boxed processed foods. The exceptions to this rule are brown rice, quinoa, oatmeal, and whole-grain bread. All of those should be staples of your diet.

SAMPLE DIET:

These are not precise recipes, simply suggestions.

DAY 1	DAY 2
Meal 1: 6 egg whites plus 2 whole scrambled eggs; 2 cups oatmeal with ½ cup raspberries; 8 ounces skim milk; 1 apple	**Meal 1:** Protein shake with 16 ounces skim milk, 2 scoops protein powder, ½ cup organic naturally flavored yogurt, 1 banana, and 1 cup frozen strawberries; 1 cup oatmeal
Meal 2: 1 scoop vanilla protein powder mixed with 1 cup fat-free cottage cheese and ½ cup blueberries; 2 baked potatoes; 1 cup raw broccoli; 1 tablespoon flaxseed oil	**Meal 2:** Omelet with 6 eggs with diced chicken, low-fat cheese, tomatoes, peppers, and onions
Meal 3: 2 grilled chicken breasts; spinach salad with peppers, onions, tomatoes, cucumbers, and apples with 1½ tablespoons olive oil and vinegar; 1 cup quinoa	**Meal 3:** 3 pieces tuna sashimi; 3 pieces salmon sashimi; seaweed salad
Meal 4: 6 ounces ground beef (93 percent lean); 2 cups steamed veggies	**Meal 4:** Post-workout shake
Meal 5: Post-workout shake	**Meal 5:** 16-ounce steak; 2 sweet potatoes; 2 cups steamed vegetables; ½ cup blueberries
Meal 6: 2 tuna sushi rolls; chicken with vegetables and brown rice	**Meal 6:** 1 can tuna; 1 cup brown rice; ½ cup black beans; mixed green salad with 2 tablespoons olive oil and vinegar; 1 apple
Meal 7: Spinach omelet made with 4 whole eggs	**Meal 7:** 1 cup fat-free or low-fat cottage cheese; 1 cup steamed green beans; 1 tablespoon flaxseed oil; 1 tablespoon hemp oil; 1 peach

Now, let's finish off with a some advanced tips to make you the best competitor you can be.

Making Weight the Right Way

As I mentioned at the start of this chapter, dehydration is the worst way to lose weight. I strongly recommend that you lose noncontractile body fat instead of your body's water stores. Your muscles are approximately 72 percent water. Dehydration of even a mere 2 percent will significantly decrease your strength, speed, and endurance. Now, let's suppose hypothetically that you are trying to move down one weight class, you have lost all the body fat that you can lose, and you still have a few last-minute pounds to drop. No problem. Below are some methods that will help you drop a few pounds of water weight before your weigh-in. These methods are quite safe, and furthermore, they should not adversely affect your performance. Before you do this, however, you must ask yourself a few questions. When is your weigh-in? Is it the day of the fight, or the day before the fight? If it's the day of the fight, how many hours prior to the fight is it? The answers to these questions are crucial in determining how much water weight you can lose and then rehydrate after weigh-in.

I want you to calculate your rehydration to be at a rate of 2 pounds per hour. So, for example, if your weigh-in is two hours prior to the fight, you can replenish 4 pounds of water in that time. Obviously, if the weigh-in is the day prior to the fight, you have much more flexibility. This is common in professional boxing.

A week prior to weigh-in, drink exactly 1 ounce of water per pound of body weight each day. There are, of course, cases in which a greater water intake would be appropriate. For instance, in a very hot climate, you can drink slightly more water. Or if the week prior to the fight is a rest week, you can drink slightly less. Either way, make sure that whatever the amount is, it is accounted for, measured, and recorded. You'll need this information later in the week as you begin to decrease your water intake.

Two days prior to weigh-in, cut your initial water intake by half. The next day (one day prior to weigh-in), cut your intake by half again. Thus, on the day before weigh-in, your intake should be one fourth of what it was at the beginning of the week.

Note: This decreased water intake should be safe, since most athletes are resting a few days prior to their fight. Thus, since you should be working out minimally, if at all, your water requirement will not be as high, and thus there should be almost no risk of dehydration.

The day of your weigh-in, only have small sips of water, just to keep your mouth wet.

Immediately after your weigh-in, you'll begin the replenishment process. Start off with a bottle of Pedialyte (available in drugstores, where it is sold as a rehydration formula for children) and a pinch of salt. Return to your normal diet. In addition, take 99 milligrams of potassium per hour and a multi-mineral containing 1000 milligrams of calcium and 500 milligrams of magnesium per day to prevent cramping and to replenish electrolytes (take this with food). And, of course, most important, drink lots of water! Specifically, drink 32 ounces of water per hour. This should guarantee that you gain back 2 pounds of water per hour. Of course, if you didn't lose that much water or you have a lot of time between weigh-in and your competition, you don't need to drink quite as much. Remember, the goal is to be rehydrated and well rested but not bloated.

In cases where you only have two hours between your weigh-in and your fight, have your Pedialyte and salt immediately after weigh-in, then 30 minutes later, have a liquid meal containing an MRP (meal-replacement powder) and some added maltodextrin (.25 grams per pound of body weight). With this meal, take your multi-mineral mentioned above, and also continue to drink 32 ounces of water per hour.

Water Intake

To prevent dehydration, it is best to drink water throughout the day, even when you're not thirsty. At the onset of thirst, the athlete is already approximately 2 percent dehydrated. Studies have shown that runners who are 2 percent dehydrated suffer a 6 to 8 percent reduction in performance, which suggests that hydration is a crucial element in training and performance.

To ensure that you don't fall prey to even slight dehydration, drink a minimum of .5 ounces of water per pound of body weight every day. Again, this is a minimal amount, and more may be required during intense training phases or in particularly hot and humid climates. Again, we are talking about pure, clear water. Not iced tea, not coffee, not beer! As a general guideline, your urine should be clear and odorless. If it isn't, you probably need to increase your water intake.

I hope that you take all of this information to heart. The work that you put in to a proper diet and training regimen will make all the difference in the world on competition day.

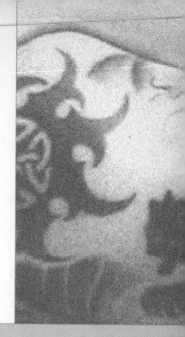

7 SUPPLEMENTS: SUBSTANCE AND THE SCAMS

These days it seems that just about every famous mixed martial artist has a supplement-endorsement deal. Every combat sports magazine you read is filled with supplement ads promising to make you stronger, richer, smarter! A number of supplement companies have even claimed their products to be steroid replacements, just as good as steroids, or even better than steroids. This is all complete B.S. There is no supplement in the world that can replace or compare with steroids. There is also no supplement in the world that can make up for poor training techniques and a crappy diet. The way to improve your strength, speed, and endurance is through hard work, proper training, and a lot of eating. If you do that, you don't need steroids anyway. Believe me, you can make mind-blowing gains without steroids if you eat right and train hard. I have even trained former steroid users who got better results using my training techniques and nutritional recommendations than they ever did on the juice. Steroids work—don't get me wrong—but there are inherent dangers associated with them that just aren't worth the risk.

Another thing you should know is that many of the magazines that are promoting these supplements are owned by supplement companies or the magazine publishers are heavy investors in the supplement industry. I couldn't believe it when I learned this information many years ago. But along with shameless promotion and dirty marketing techniques, most supplement companies do whatever they can to cut costs and increase their profit margins—and they do this by misleading you.

I learned firsthand how this works a few years back when I decided to formulate my own batch of protein powder. I used the same lab some of the biggest-name companies use, and I was stunned by what I learned.

When it comes to formulating a supplement, you get what you pay for. What this means is that companies choose how much money they want to spend on a particular product, and that decision dictates the quality of that product. For example, when formulating my own protein powder, I brought some of the most popular brands to the lab and said that we wanted ours to have a similar taste, texture, and quality. Well, the taste and texture would be no problem, but it would hardly be a *quality* product if we copied the leaders of the supplement industry.

The lab ran tests on the batches of the popular protein powders that we brought in, and we were told by one of the chemists that he, and I quote, "wouldn't allow his dog to eat this crap." He went on to explain that the company had chosen such cheap ingredients that the product probably was doing more harm than good. He told us that what this company was selling for thirty or forty dollars per bottle actually cost them under five bucks to make!

As we were walking through the lab, we noticed several bottles of what has since become the most popular protein powder on the market because of its incredible taste. I'm sure you know the one; it's loaded with sugar and has the fat content of a double cheeseburger. The chemist we were working with had actually worked with the owners of that company on formulating the product and told us that when developing their protein powder all they cared about was that it "taste like Häagen-Dazs." They didn't care what kind of garbage ingredients were included to achieve the taste as long as people loved the product. Apparently, they had the right idea because it went on to be a huge seller. The sad part is that people don't know that what they are consuming is pure sewage. Even carefully reading the label doesn't give you an honest idea of what these shysters are packing into each container—while the label will tell you some of the primary ingredients, it won't list the fillers, which frequently include ash and all kinds of other junk.

From this experience we learned that most protein powders are made with the lowest-quality protein available and that they only put in a pinch of some of the popular "high-tech" proteins brazenly touted on the label. If the bottle contains even 1 teaspoon of the advertised ingredient, say casein, they can claim it on the label and they can't get in trouble for lying. Deceptive, isn't it?

It is entirely possible that most of the powder that you scoop into your blender each morning is mainly cheap filler. And most protein powders contain up to three packets of aspartame per scoop! For those of you who don't know, artificial sweeteners have been shown in numerous studies to be dangerous to your health. While many of the damning studies have been conducted outside of the United States, the results still are cause for real concern. Several studies have shown aspartame to be related to birth defects, memory loss, and decreased functioning of the sexual organs. None of those sound the least bit appealing to me, especially the not being able to have sex part . . . but then again, if I couldn't remember it, maybe it wouldn't be so bad.

Since reading these studies, I have sworn off aspartame. I will eat real sugar over fake any day of the week; aspartame is just not worth the risk. While you're reading labels, make sure to check for the presence of aspartame.

More Useless Crap

Believe it or not, there actually are a few supplements that I believe may be of use to you. But before we get into those, I want to briefly mention a few more of today's most popular supplement scams to help you save your money.

Acetyl-L-Carnitine

This supplement was first prescribed for patients with memory loss and other cognitive dysfunction. Like many other supplements, its makers claim that it has been shown to improve testosterone levels and energy production, boost the immune system, and so on and so on. It worked its way into bodybuilding circles because its manufacturers claimed that it was a great performance booster if taken in very large, and quite expensive, doses. Thousands of bodybuilders have since proven it to be worthless.

Alpha-Lipoic Acid

This compound is touted to improve insulin sensitivity and help users metabolize and store carbohydrates more efficiently. In the late 90s it became popular to take this supplement with a post-workout drink or on carb-load days. The supplement was said to work by sucking up all the carbs straight into your muscles and presto . . . you would be hyooooge!!! Not really. In fact, nothing happened. Ever.

Ashwaganda

This little-known herb from India was purported to increase sperm count and testosterone levels dramatically. It was also supposed to increase your strength in the gym dramatically if taken in extremely high doses. I went through ten bottles of this garbage in one month before I realized I had been duped—I didn't experience the slightest increase in strength gains. Unfortunately, I suckered a few close friends into emptying their wallets with me, and they were upset with me to say the least.

Chitosan

According to the label, chitosan should be taken before you eat a high-fat meal. The claim is that it somehow will suck up all the fat in the food and eliminate it from your body before it is absorbed and stored as body fat. You can get up off the floor when you finish laughing. If this were possible, we could all live on pizza and cheeseburgers and have the physiques of Olympic sprinters. Obviously, this is one of the more blatant rip-offs in supplement history.

Colostrum

The sucker story behind colostrum is a great one—it could get almost anyone to try it at least once. Colostrum is secreted in mother's milk and is highly anabolic (the condition under which muscle grows). The rap is that there is no period in our life span when we grow faster than in those first few months after birth, when we're being nourished by our mother's milk. Supplement manufacturers thought that if they could bottle this anabolic substance it would be the greatest compound to ever hit the market. I have to admit that I fell for this one as well. I gave it a shot but quickly wised up and only wasted money on one bottle. At the time I knew many people who bought several bottles only to realize, months later, that they had been scammed yet again when the product did none of what it promised. You have to admit, though, it was a great sales pitch.

Forskolin

This herb has been promoted as both a fat-loss supplement and a testosterone booster. It is neither. Enough said.

Ipriflavone

This is a compound derived from plants that is intended for use on osteoporosis patients. Somehow someone came up with the idea that since it was shown to help prevent bone loss, it also would magically prevent muscle loss. And if taken in high enough doses, it might even increase muscle gains. Now I know this sounds ridiculous, but I gave it a shot. I mean I really gave it a shot. I was taking bottles of this back in the late 90s. As usual, I scammed some friends into hopping on the bandwagon with me, and a month later they all wanted to kill me. Suckered again . . .

Myostatin Suppressors

This supplement may take the cake as the worst scam of all time. Myostatin suppressors sum up the entire supplement industry and all of its dirty little lies and scumbag tactics. To understand why myostatin-suppressing supplements rank so low in my book, you need to know the story behind them.

The hype for this supplement was amazing, and the ads all told the same story: You'd see a picture of an incredibly muscular cow that reportedly had its myostatin gene blocked or never had one (I don't remember the precise details). To a large extent, our genes control our ability to gain muscle and lose fat, and all of us eventually will reach a point where we've reached our full potential. The gene responsible for stopping muscle growth and increasing fat storage is . . . you guessed it, the myostatin gene.

Now, if only there were a way to somehow suppress myostatin, we all would be able to grow without limits and get as lean as we wanted to. If this were possible, we'd soon see 400-pound monsters everywhere.

I don't want to bore you with the rest of the story, because by now you all have surely realized what a horrible lie this is and how it is downright negligent to perpetrate such falsehoods on the public. Obviously, there is no possible way to grow infinitely or to suppress the mysotatin gene. Are we really supposed to believe that supplement company owners, many of whom are ex–drug dealers and convicts, somehow did what the world's most brilliant doctors and scientists could never do? If there are really minds this brilliant out there, why are they not curing cancer or AIDS? Instead, they are showing bodybuilders how to turn into real-life-sized versions of the Incredible Hulk? Give me a break. Anyone who was ever involved in the creation or promotion of this supplement should be deeply ashamed of themselves.

Taurine

This amino acid was meant to be taken with other supplements such as creatine and glutamine for a "volumizing" effect, meaning that it would cause great swelling inside the muscle, which would lead to a more anabolic state. If you want swelling, drink a gallon of salt water . . . or watch a Jenna Jameson DVD. Otherwise steer clear of the taurine aisle.

Theophylline

This compound was added to certain fat-loss supplements back in the early 90s and was supposed to aid in fat loss but ended up causing more harm than good. Over the last several years there has been considerable evidence to show that the use of this compound is actually quite dangerous. The drug's legitimate use is for the treatment of serious lung disease, and because of its serious side effects, it must be carefully monitored to avoid toxicity. Steer clear.

Yohimbine

This was promoted as both a fat-loss supplement and libido booster. According to the hype, yohimbine increases blood flow to the extremities, meaning that it will both improve erections and somehow increase localized fat burning. In addition to the pill version, a topical yohimbine cream was also marketed. This was touted as an aid for promoting fat loss in those stubborn areas, such as the hamstrings and glutes. This is one I've not tried, but from what I've heard both the supplement and the cream were useless.

ZMA

That people ever got bamboozled into paying thirty bucks for a bottle of zinc and magnesium is completely baffling to me. ZMA is zinc and magnesium! These compounds are available in every pharmacy and supermarket in the country for about five bucks a bottle or less. But sometime back in the late 90s, a guy by the name of Victor Conte was studying the effects of zinc and magnesium deficiencies in people and was convinced that he had to do something about the problem.

The fact of the matter is that hardly anyone is deficient in zinc. It's like living in Florida and saying you're deficient in sunlight. But Conte found a study that showed that Navy seals had low testosterone levels after rigorous training. Low testosterone is often the result of overtraining, so no surprise here. But in this study, the problem apparently was fixed with zinc.

Bizarrely, Conte also concluded that these Navy Seals were deficient in magnesium as well. While magnesium deficiencies are more common than zinc deficiencies, it's not like this is the kind of problem that is running rampant and ruining peoples' lives.

But for Conte and his company, BALCO Labs, these deficiency "problems" presented a huge sales and marketing opportunity. For only through their "special" combination of zinc and magnesium could you jack up your testosterone levels and build muscle like crazy. And why the magnesium-zinc combo? According to Conte, if you take zinc with any other nutrients, it won't be absorbed. That is why you needed his supplement and why you couldn't get your zinc from a basic multivitamin. He forgot just one small piece of critical information, though. Zinc is naturally present in many of the foods we eat and is always consumed with other nutrients. Human beings have been able to absorb zinc just fine since the beginning of time. This has never, ever been a problem.

So needless to say, the "genius" idea of putting zinc and magnesium in a bottle and calling it an anabolic compound never quite panned out. In fact, it was among the top scams in supplement history only because of how hard it was pushed. But to this day, people are still buying ZMA and getting suckered into thinking that paying thirty dollars for a five-dollar bottle of zinc and magnesium somehow will help them build muscle.

What Works

By now you might have guessed that I am not a big fan of supplements, and I'm sure you can see why. Most supplements are completely useless and some are not just useless, but dangerous as well.

However, there are a few supplements that are worth trying. But please remember one important fact: A supplement is just that. Supplements cannot take the place of either a decent diet or a good training program, and there is not a supplement in creation that can replicate the effects of steroids. It's impossible, has never happened, will never happen. If your diet and training are in order and you have been working diligently at both for at least a year or two, then you might want to give a few of the supplements below a try.

Multivitamins

A good multivitamin and mineral supplement is nothing more than insurance against a less-than-perfect diet. Let's face it, few guys eat all the fruits and vegetables that they should on a regular basis. That is where taking a multivitamin can be of benefit to you. There is nothing magical about a multivitamin, but it may be beneficial to your overall health. Besides, if you're not healthy, you can't train, and if you can't train, you can't make progress. I always recommend eating a healthy diet rich in fruits and vegetables as your first option, but if you can't do that, then a multivitamin is a decent idea.

Note: you do not need high-dose vitamins. Don't get scammed into wasting your money on taking tons of vitamins and minerals every day. The reality is that vitamin and mineral deficiencies are rare in our country. Furthermore, no matter what anyone promises you, megadoses of vitamins or minerals will not enhance performance to any noticeable degree. In fact the most benefit you'll get from high doses is very expensive, vitamin-packed piss.

Omega-3 Fish Oils

Omega-3 fish oils are one of the few supplements I would say are musthaves. They have a wide array of health benefits, including decreased cholesterol levels and blood pressure. And of great interest to those trying to get big and perform on a high level, they also have the following benefits:

- Reduction of joint pain
- Increased energy levels
- Decreased inflammation throughout the entire body
- Improved functioning of the immune system
- Increased strength levels
- Increased testosterone levels
- Increased levels of HGH (human growth hormone)
- Increased oxygen delivery to the cells during workouts
- Decreased body fat
- Increased insulin sensitivity

Take 6 to 12 grams a day spread evenly over the course of five or six meals. Be sure to get a good pharmaceutical-grade brand of fish oils; otherwise you could be doing yourself more harm than good. The cheap stuff is filled with pollutants and usually is rancid before you even open the bottle.

Protein Powder

For most of us, it is quite difficult to consume our daily requirement of protein by eating nothing but real, solid food. Getting in 200-plus grams of protein a day even when you're eating chicken, eggs, fish, and beef is tough—especially when you are busy training. Obviously, if you can meet your daily protein requirements by just eating real food, then that is definitely the way to go. Food beats supplements every day of the week. But if you can't, then a protein shake will help you get there. Try not to rely on them, though, and instead eat as much real food as you can, using shakes to make up the deficit.

When shopping for protein powder, look for formulas that contain a good blend of whey, casein, and milk protein isolate. Pure whey protein is not great to consume on its own because it is very rapidly digested and has a very high glycemic index, which can lead to fat gain. If you have no choice, make sure to mix your whey with some skim milk and/or cottage cheese to get more of a more-complex protein blend and slow down the insulin response of the whey.

I prefer to avoid artificial sweeteners, so I opt for natural protein powder that doesn't contain any artificial ingredients. These brands are often harder to find but are worth tracking down. As I mentioned, the studies on aspartame and other artificial sweeteners have convinced me that these products are best avoided. If I'm going to drink unhealthy beverages, I'll stick to vodka and beer . . .

Your protein shake should contain a healthy mix of protein, fiber, and essential fats. Some protein powders contain fibers and good fats, but most don't. The best way to include these is to add them yourself. You can doctor up your shake with fruit, peanut butter, cottage cheese, nuts, and any number of healthy ingredients.

Most days I make my shake with organic skim milk, cottage cheese or yogurt, frozen berries, a tablespoon of natural peanut butter or olive oil, and a scoop or two of natural protein powder. If you are on the run or don't have access to a blender, you can simply mix some protein powder with skim milk or water and eat a handful of nuts to get some good fat in.

Creatine Monohydrate

If you would like to experiment with another supplement that may help in your muscle-building quest, give creatine monohydrate a try. Creatine is found naturally in red meat; however, you would have to eat an inordinate amount to derive any performance-enhancing benefits. This is one supplement that has been shown in countless studies to deliver results. Creatine has been used by athletes for at least fourteen years without any negative side effects. Some studies have reported a 5 to 15 percent increase in maximal strength and power from creatine usage. Most users also report significant weight gain due to greater storage of intracellular fluids. This is not true muscle gain, but it is not just water retention either. Water retention is held outside of the cells, while the fluid stored with creatine is intracellular. Intramuscular stores of creatine have been shown to increase by as much as 50 percent after five days of creatine supplementation.

The weight gained while using creatine increases the surface area of the muscles, which increases the potential for strength. Many users also report far greater pumps (the ego-boosting, skin-tightening feeling you get when your muscles are engorged with blood after a few sets) while using creatine. It has also been shown to have a lactic acid–buffering effect, meaning that it delays the burn you feel in the middle of a set that makes you want to drop the weights. As a result, the set may feel easier to you than you had anticipated, and you may be able to squeeze out a few more reps. Another benefit of creatine is that it can delay the sense of fatigue over the course of a workout, allowing you to complete later sets (which you normally wouldn't be able to push yourself very hard on) with a greater intensity than you would if you weren't using it.

Finally, creatine recently has been shown to also improve overall health and brain function. Two huge benefits, if you ask me. The normal recommended dose is 3 to 5 grams a day. Most experts recommend a loading phase of 15 to 25 grams a day for 5 to 7 days, but this is not completely necessary. You can simply start taking 3 to 5 grams a day. You will experience similar results, although it probably will take longer to reach a therapeutic dose. Contrary to some recommendations, you don't have to cycle off creatine. There are no advantages to doing so and no known negative effects from long-term usage.

You may be confused by the myriad brands on the shelf. My advice is that you should stick to regular, plain, old-fashioned creatine—it works as well as any of the fancy, higher-priced stuff out there today. Skip the brands hyping added high-tech ingredients, and those claiming that you will get 20 percent better results. This is all just marketing hype. For years most experts advised taking creatine with a high-sugar beverage, such as grape juice, to speed the creatine into your system. But this "fact" has been disproved. Stick with plain micronized creatine. Mix it in a hot beverage such as green tea or in your post-workout shake, and you will be fine.

Having said all of that, I should point out that I haven't seen a single person get mind-blowing results from creatine supplementation. Although many swear by it and just as many others get great placebo effects from it, creatine is just a supplement, and supplements can provide you with only a slight edge above what you could achieve without them. If your diet and training are in check and you are really at the top of your game, you could give creatine a try and hope to achieve a slight edge.

Caffeine

My favorite pre-workout supplement is really not a supplement at all; it's just plain old caffeine. Before a big workout, you will be hard-pressed to find a supplement that gives any more of a kick than a good strong dose of caffeine. I recommend saving caffeine for when you really need it, no more than 2 to 3 times a week at the very most. Using it more often than that will negate its effects. People who get addicted to caffeine and use it on a regular basis suffer from a reduction in insulin sensitivity. This means that they cannot tolerate carbohydrates as well and are more likely to get fat from eating them. Chronic use of caffeine at doses higher than 200 milligrams a day also burns out the adrenal glands, making it harder to get or stay lean.

A better everyday choice than coffee or caffeine pills such as Vivarin, a favorite with many gym rats, is green tea. The health benefits and antioxidant properties of green tea are well known, and the caffeine content is significantly lower than that of coffee. It provides just enough caffeine to give you a slight kick without overstimulating your central nervous system. A cup of hot green tea consumed right before training also can help raise core temperature and decrease the amount of warm-up time needed.

Mixed Greens Products

Most of us will never eat enough fruits—and especially vegetables—no matter how hard we try, so supplementing with a mixed greens product is a great idea. This is basically a powdered blend of a wide variety of fruits and vegetables. UFC legend Randy Couture even has his own such product, called Life Force, which is made with crushed greens.

Post-Workout Drinks

If you read fitness magazines, you've probably seen all the hype about consuming post-workout shakes IMMEDIATELY after training. Many guys have become convinced that if they don't inhale a fast-acting shake the instant they finish their last set, they'll start shrinking immediately. Clearly, this is nonsense. It doesn't make the slightest bit of difference in the real world.

There have been lots of studies that suggest that post-workout drinks are highly effective in helping recovery and improving performance. The problem is that all of the studies were done on endurance athletes in a fasted state and not on weight-training athletes. There is a huge difference between doing an all-day triathlon and doing a forty-minute workout consisting of twelve sets of presses, rows, and squats. I can only guess that your body probably will be more starved for nutrients after a triathlon but, like I said, it's just a guess.

Having said that, I still think it's a good idea to have a post-workout shake right after training for the simple reason that you probably haven't eaten in at least two hours, and by the time you leave the gym, shower, and get home (or wherever you eat), it could be another hour. A post-workout shake simply allows you to ingest more calories while also replenishing your glycogen stores, which will be depleted after training (although nowhere near as much as some supplement manufacturers would like you to believe). It has also been established that the stress hormone cortisol can be elevated after a hard workout. Protein and carb drinks have been shown to bring cortisol levels back to normal. That is definitely a positive benefit. And, as a combat athlete, your body takes a real beating—a post-workout drink can speed your recovery.

Can you get the same effects from drinking some fat-free chocolate milk? Quite possibly. But if you choose to buy a premixed post-workout concoction I have no problem with that. It certainly isn't going to hurt you, and it isn't just another scam based completely on lies.

Thermogenics, aka Fat Burners

These dietary supplements are typically made of caffeine and herbs and are used for their stimulant effects. I only recommend fat burners during the last three to four weeks of a very long, strict fat-loss diet when you've gotten down to single-digit body fat and are looking to go even lower. But, as I've stressed before, your diet and training should be your primary focus. There are no shortcuts.

One of the problems with relying on fat burners is that you can get addicted to them. Many people like the energy boost, and it gives them an excuse to be less strict with their diet while still staying lean. But if you use fat burners for too long, your adrenal glands eventually will burn out. Adrenal fatigue is very difficult to recover from and takes some time. You'll feel sluggish, and you'll find it difficult to lose fat in the future. Still enthused about trying fat burners?

In the old days, most "therms" consisted of caffeine and ephedrine. Since ephedrine is no longer available over the counter, many companies have come up with replacement ingredients, some effective, some not so effective. If you opt to use therms, be smart and conservative and NEVER use them more than twice a year, and restrict each cycle to no more than three or four weeks.

Neurotransmitter Formulas, aka Brain Stimulants

There are several supplement combinations that consist of a group of herbs including ginkgo biloba, DMAE, L-tyrosine, and phosphatidyl-choline. These formulas are intended to improve the mind-muscle connection, as well as increase concentration, memory, coordination, and endurance. Users also report an improved sense of well-being and lower perceived levels of exertion. One of the main benefits of these supplements is that they give you increased energy and focus without giving you that jittery feeling that you get from caffeine or ephedrine; hence the term *brain stimulant*.

I have experimented with many of these combinations and have found them to be useful and effective before a workout. Several of my clients have experienced similar results and now use these supplements on a regular basis. One of the added benefits is that some of these herbs may help regenerate the central nervous system after intense training. While this is debatable, it can't hurt to try them.

I'd also like to point out that 3,000 milligrams of L-tyrosine, a brain stimulant, taken with 200 milligrams of caffeine before training, is an extremely potent stack and is probably the most effective pre-workout combination I have ever tried.

The Bottom Line on Supplements

That short list above is all you'll ever really need when it comes to supplements. The fact is, you don't even need most of those either; plenty of people have done just fine without them. While there are a few other supplements that may in fact "do something," I don't feel that most of them are even worth mentioning.

Now that I have exposed the supplement industry and all of its dirty lies, I truly hope that you are ready to stop throwing your money away and destroying your health with all of this useless garbage that these hucksters are trying to sell you. The fact of the matter is that these soulless bastards will do anything that they can to get you to part with your money. You now have the knowledge to stand up to the corporations and tell them you're not falling for their lies anymore.

A supplement is just a supplement; never forget that important fact. Personally, the only thing I take regularly are fish oil and some natural protein powder. I have also known plenty of the biggest and strongest guys in the world (some of whom are my close friends) who don't take supplements either. Supplements are far from necessary, and as you know by now, they definitely aren't the magic bullet many advertisers make them out to be. You can achieve outstanding results through hard training and a well-rounded diet.

Everyone would love a magic bullet, so I know that much of this information will disappoint many of you. But let me leave you with something positive. There actually is an amazing muscle-building source so powerful it will blow you away. It is responsible for every ounce of lean tissue that you gain. Some might even say that its effects are druglike.

It's called food. Eat ample quantities of it in the right ratios and from the right sources and you will build muscle and burn fat.

So the next time you are in search of more muscle and less body fat, go eat a steak and potato. It will do more for you than any pills or powder ever could.

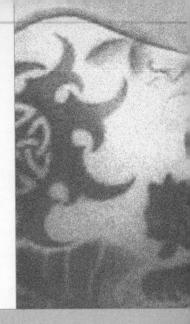

8 PICKING UP THE PIECES: RECOVERY AND REGENERATION

A COMBAT ATHLETE USUALLY PUTS HIS BODY THROUGH HELL IN an effort to be the best at what he does. The actual practice sessions coupled with weight-training workouts and extra conditioning take a real toll. Your ability to recover from all these stresses can make the difference between a champion and a loser. Your goal is to progress, both in terms of strength and ability, and to remain injury-free. To do so you have to use every recovery method you can. In this chapter, I'm going to give you the top recovery methods I use with all my athletes.

1. Drink a post-workout shake. Immediately after training, consume a mix of high-glycemic carbs and rapidly absorbed protein (see Guideline #5 in Chapter 6 for specifics). This drink should contain a 2-to-1 ratio of carbs to protein. A 200-pound man would consume roughly 80 grams of carbs and 40 grams of protein. The formula for you might be a little different, based on insulin sensitivity, body-fat levels, and

- **Should I worry about electrolyte depletion?**

- If you are training for more than one hour (especially under hot and humid conditions), you obviously want to drink water throughout your workout, but after the first hour also begin sipping Gatorade or a similar electrolyte-replenishing drink. Gauge this according to how you feel during the workout—the goal here is to avoid electrolyte loss.

- The primary electrolytes we are concerned with here are sodium, potassium, and magnesium. Common symptoms of electrolyte loss are muscle cramping, weakness, fatigue, and nausea. If any of these symptoms become severe, you should cease your workout immediately and replenish electrolytes and fluids aggressively.

training volume, but the 2-to-1 ratio is a good start. Consuming this shake will help reduce your cortisol levels and will shuttle nutrients to your muscles and so begin the recovery process.

2. Use cold therapy. Most athletes shy away from using cold modalities (such as ice or ice baths) as a recovery method. But those athletes who do see the benefits quickly welcome it as part of their daily routine. To be honest, the first time you try an ice bath, you'll find it extremely intense and very uncomfortable. No one really likes to stick their feet (or other body parts) in a bucket of ice water. However, in my experience, cold therapy is one of the best ways to quickly slow down the inflammation process and combat the muscle and joint pain that can occur from hard daily training.

I recommend the following four cold-therapy methods:

Ice Bags I always tell my athletes to strap a bag of crushed ice on their sore and painful areas immediately after their training session. Do this even before jumping into a hot shower. Out of the gym, into the ice. For sore shoulders, elbows, knees, ankles, or just about any other body part, use ice bags as part of your daily routine—you won't be sorry. Get some crushed ice, place it into a zip-top baggie, and put it right on your skin. Ice for no longer than 20 minutes at a time with at least an hour in between icings. If you are on the go, use an Ace wrap or some kind of sleeve to keep the ice in place.

Ice Baths This is a more extreme method of cold therapy but also one of the best. I usually use this on my athletes who have chronic pain or inflammation in their feet, ankles, and/or lower legs. (e.g., shin splints) and even some who have bad knees. Fill a large bucket or bathtub with ice and water. Place your foot, ankle, or leg into the water. Be forewarned, this is not easy. I have watched some of the toughest SOBs in the business cry and scream like babies for the first few minutes after immersion. Stay tough and wait for about 3 to 5 minutes. After that, you will go numb in the area and it won't bother you much at all. I have seen athletes with extremely inflamed joints and other painful conditions come out of an ice bath feeling like brand-new. Again, no more than 20 minutes in the ice bath.

Ice Massage This is yet another intense form of cold therapy but a very good one. If you have a very sore or inflamed smaller area, like the tip of your shoulder, patellar tendons, or elbow, give the ice massage a try. Just get a few small paper cups, fill them with water, and place them in the freezer. Once they are frozen, take one out, peel around the top of the cup, and your ice massage is ready to go. Moving quickly, rub the ice around the affected area in a small circle, never stopping the motion. Do this for about 5 to 10 minutes, no more. This therapy is quite intense; you may even see a small welt form over the affected area. But don't worry—it's just a reaction from the ice. Simply stop and throw your ice away. You are done for that session. I have used ice massage with my athletes very successfully over the years and have seen incredible results.

Cold Shower This is perhaps the most controversial of the cold therapies. Many people believe that cold showers (when I say cold, I mean ice-cold) don't do much except torture the person taking them. However, as with most things, people are different and have different opinions. Some of my athletes love to take a very cold shower after an intense workout. It seems to invigorate them, take away some of the aches and pains that were induced during training, and help their overall recovery. Others think it makes things worse. Either way, it is something else you can try and see how it works for you.

3. Use heat therapy. Once you're home, showered, and calmed down, heat can be a great way to help relax different body parts. It's also great for reducing pain and inflammation. Word of warning: Heat should NEVER be used on an acute injury. For acute injuries, use ice. You can heat safely a few days later. Below are my favorite methods:

Hot packs Whether an electric heating pad or a moist hot pack, hot packs are great to use over areas of the body. I tend to use hot packs with my athletes who suffer from stiff, nagging injuries that don't seem to go away. Twenty to thirty minutes of heat on the right place can make all the difference in easing aches and pains.

Hot Baths Like cold or ice-water baths, hot baths can have a tremendous effect on recovery and, let's face it, are much more comfortable than cold. A hot bath, Jacuzzi hot tub, or spa will do the trick. Try not to stay in for more than 30 to 40 minutes at a time. You can become dehydrated pretty fast sitting in a hot bath, and hydration is extremely important. Make sure to drink water while you are in the tub to keep

---

TIPS FROM THE CAGE

- **How can you tell if you're overtraining, and how do you avoid doing so?**

- This is a tough one, because everyone is different and what may kill me may be the perfect amount of training for you. The easiest way to tell if you are overtraining is just to watch your rate of progress. If you are continually making progress, then you are not overtraining. If your progress is slow or halted, then the most likely cause is overtraining. You could also be undereating and/or not utilizing proper recovery methods, but that still equates to overtraining. Another thing to look at is your motivation level. If you are no longer motivated to train and feel sluggish and weak, you most likely are overtraining. An elevated morning heart rate, a decrease in appetite, and an inability to sleep are other signs to look out for.

   As far as avoiding overtraining goes, if you follow my guidelines for training and recovery, you should be okay. Make sure to take a complete week off every 8 to 12 weeks. Another important thing: Do not push yourself to failure and/or beyond on every set you do in the gym. There should be a week-to-week progression of how much effort you put into your sets during each 4-week block of training. On week 1 you are just being introduced to the exercises and establishing a feel for them and the kinds of weights you are going to use. You should not come close to failure on any of these sets. On week 2, you can push it a little more, but still don't go to failure on any sets. When you get to week 3, you can really push yourself and just about hit failure on every set. Make sure you complete each rep with good form, though, and don't actually fail on any given set or rep. Save that for the last week, when you will go for broke, try to set new personal bets, and push yourself as hard as you possibly can. If you follow this progression you definitely will be at a much lower risk for overtraining.

yourself from getting dehydrated. I tell my wrestlers to hit the hot tub each night before they go to bed. It helps relax them, calms down muscle spasms, and always seems to lead to a great night's sleep. Remember, rest is one of the big keys for total recovery.

4. Do not drop carbohydrate intake too low.   Although low-carb diets are in vogue these days, this is not an optimal approach for a hard-training athlete. Even if you need to lose a good amount of body fat, you still should be consuming at least 150 to 200 grams of carbs a day. Dropping carbs drastically will slow down your thyroid and testosterone production and cause you to lose size and strength. To maximize your recovery, you must keep a decent amount of carbs in your diet. As a hard-training combat athlete, your energy-system demands are off the charts, so you need an adequate amount of carbohydrates for recovery. Focus on natural, organic sources such as fruits, vegetables (including sweet potatoes and white potatoes), legumes, and oats.

5. Take naps.   Naps are a great way to speed up your recovery. During sleep, your body releases growth hormone and repairs the damage that has been done to your muscles during intense workouts. A 20- to 60-minute nap once a day is a great way to make faster progress. If you are training two to three times a day, as many combat athletes are (conditioning in the morning, practice in the afternoon, weight training at night), naps are an absolute necessity if you want to maximize your performance.

6. Sleep eight to ten hours a night.   As mentioned above, when you are sleeping, you are growing bigger and stronger and repairing the damage done to your muscles during hard workouts. Without sufficient sleep, your results will be less than optimal. If you have difficulty sleeping, please do not ignore this section. There are many books that deal with improving the quality of your sleep, and it is highly recommended that you read one. But here are a few tips that can help you achieve better sleeping habits:

- Go to bed and get up at the same time every day.
- Unwind for an hour before bed. During this time you should be doing nothing but relaxing. Reading is okay here, as long as it is not something that gets your mind overstimulated—fiction or something that is not at all related to anything you do is usually best here.
- Make your room as dark as possible. One study showed that even a tiny light shining directly on the back of a patient's leg negatively affected sleep quality.
- Avoid alcohol, as it can negatively affect the quality of your sleep.
- Don't eat too much protein immediately before bed. Protein contains tyrosine, an amino acid that sends a signal to your brain to become more alert. Having a huge protein meal before bed is a good way to ensure that you will be up for a while.
- Don't drink too much water before bed. This is another way of disruping your sleep quality, because you will be up visiting the bathroom when you should be sleeping and recovering.
- Keep your bedroom slightly cool. The optimal sleeping temperature is around 68 to 70 degrees. Having your room much warmer than this also can negatively affect the quality of your sleep.

7. Stretch on your off days. This is a great way of increasing blood flow to the muscles, which helps shuttle in the nutrients necessary for optimal recovery. There is much debate on which type of stretching is best. In my opinion, you should use every method of stretching available to you, including PNF (proprioceptive neuromuscular facilitation), static, and dynamic. PNF stretching, also known as the contract-relax method, is usually done with a partner. In this style of stretching you contract the muscle you are attempting to stretch against resistance (usually applied by a partner). You should not forcefully contract the muscle but only use about 25 percent of your strength. Hold the stretch for 6 to 8 seconds and then take a deep breath while briefly relaxing the muscle and then trying to stretch it farther. You do this until you can't go any farther.

Static stretching is the way most people are used to stretching. It simply involves getting into a stretch and holding it for 30 to 60 seconds. Dynamic stretching is stretching while moving. Leg swings are an example of dynamic stretches, as are most forms of kicks. Pick up a book on stretching for a more complete discussion of this complex topic.

TIPS FROM THE CAGE

- **Should conditioning methods change during the off-season?**

- The answer to this really depends on the time of the year. If you are in the beginning of the off-season (or in the downtime between fights), you should limit your amount of conditioning. The focus during this time should be to correct any imbalances that might have developed over the course of the year. You also need to rehab any injuries and work on preventing new ones. As your training progresses, you should start to add some conditioning back about twelve weeks from the season or competition. Start with one session per week, in addition to your practices or other training sessions. As the season/event gets closer, you can add more conditioning sessions as you lower the volume of your weight training. During the final month, you will be working on your skills and practicing nearly every day, so both the strength and conditioning volume will be lowered during this time period.

Of course, the more direct answer to this question is actually a question itself. How much do you need to work on your conditioning? If it is a major weakness for you, more so than speed, strength, and even skill, then you definitely need to address this throughout the entire off-season.

Below is an example of when to schedule and integrate your conditioning workouts with the rest of your program.

Beginning of off-season:

Monday: Full-body weight training

Tuesday: Skill training

Wednesday: Full-body weight training

Thursday: Skill training

Friday: Full-body weight training

Saturday: Conditioning

Sunday: Off

Middle of off-season:

Monday: Full-body weight training

Tuesday: Skill training and conditioning

Wednesday: Full-body weight training

Thursday: Skill training

Friday: Full-body weight training

Saturday: Skill training and conditioning

Sunday: Off

End of off-season:

Monday: Full-body weight training

Tuesday: Skill training and conditioning

Wednesday: Skill training and conditioning

Thursday: Full-body weight training

Friday: Skill training and conditioning

Saturday: Skill training and optional conditioning

Sunday: Off

8. Do recovery workouts. By performing a very light, high-rep workout the day after an intense training session and getting some blood into the muscles, you can accelerate recovery. For example, the day after a heavy squat workout, your legs are likely to be very sore. Instead of doing nothing, try going for a 10-minute walk with a lightly weighted sled. Sleds are available at www.EliteFTS.com.

9. Get a massage once a week. This is a great way to relax and speed up the healing process of sore muscles. Be sure to drink lots of water in the hours following a massage to help rid the body of toxins released during the treatment. If you cannot afford a massage, you could try self-massage, or if you are lucky enough to have a girlfriend or wife who could assist you, it's always worth begging her. At the very least, you should be using a foam roller; foam rollers are cylinders that come in varying lengths and diameters and that are used to perform a kind of self-massage, breaking up scar tissue in the muscles and increasing blood flow. Foam rolling also increases flexibility and speeds muscle recovery after workouts. All you need to do is roll the affected area on the hard foam and tolerate the pressure it puts on your muscles. It can be intense at first, but consider this—the areas that hurt the most are generally the tightest and need the most attention. Rollers are available at optp.com.

10. Avoid stress. This is obviously easier said than done, but it should be noted that excessive amounts of psychological or emotional stress can wreak havoc on your results. Stress causes the body to release cortisol, a hormone that eats muscle tissue. Excessive amounts of cortisol can also cause an increase in body-fat levels, especially around the abdomen. As a combat athlete, your body already has enough stress to deal with, so do yourself a favor and don't make it worse.

11. Take a week off. Every six to twelve weeks, your body will start to break down and demand a rest. Taking a week off will allow you to get stronger and come back fresh and ready to train hard again. The older and more experienced you get, the more frequently you will need to take a week off. Many of my older athletes take a complete week off every three to four weeks. This obviously is not possible for someone who is trying to reach the highest level of combat sports, but it's a good guideline to keep in mind. Many combat athletes seriously overtrain, which has negative effects over time. Scheduling time off can help you avoid the problems associated with overtraining.

Remember, training is only half the equation. Without proper recovery techniques, your progress will never be optimal. Start using these methods today and watch your results skyrocket.

RESOURCES

For training equipment such as sleds, blast straps, ropes, and the prowler, go to www.EliteFTS.com.

For sandbags, neck harnesses, straps, and grip-training tools, go to www.IronMind.com.

For strongman equipment, visit www.TotalPerformanceSports.com or www.AtomicAthletic.com.

For plyometric boxes, hurdles, and medicine balls, go to www.Perform Better.com.

To keep a diet log online and compute your daily caloric breakdown and total intake, go to www.FitDay.com.

For foam rollers, visit www.optp.com.

INDEX